7 EXERCISE MYTHS THAT ARE KILLING AMERICANS

"Gordon Duffy has done a fantastic job of dispelling the myths supported by the mass media that give you mediocre gains at best. By showing you what really works, and the rationale behind it, he will make your quest for rapid gains in fitness levels and body composition a reality."

— Charles Poliquin,
Coach to 17 Olympic medalists & 10 world record holders

"No one could be more qualified than Gordon Duffy to teach someone how to train. If he's looking for clients, I will be his first."

— Bill Pearl,
The World's #1 Trainer

"Few experts can tell you why some of the most commonly used exercises can actually harm you. This breakthrough book gives you a really good scientifically based foundation to functional fitness with the purpose of helping your body functions last for life."

— Dr. Shu Li,
Chairman, World Anti-Aging Center, Shanghai, China

"Having trained all my life both on my own and with professional trainers, I knew I needed a different game plan as I approached fifty. I have never felt or looked better, but more importantly, I know that I am healthier and better able to manage and enjoy life for the next fifty years."

— Ash Narayan, JD, CPA, CFP®

"I've been concerned with personal fitness all my adult life. I was a long-distance runner in high school, a rower in college, and have always belonged to a gym and prided myself on being 'in shape.' Gordon has demonstrated to me that I was wasting a lot of effort, overworking muscles and joints that needed a rest and neglecting my core. Gordon's approach and techniques are like nothing I've ever been exposed to, and my time with him has definitely enriched—and probably extended—my life. Now I know what being in shape truly means."

— Larry C. Boyd,
Executive VP & General Counsel, Ingram Micro Inc.

"Like many passionate workout enthusiasts, I used conventional cardio training throughout my life for my physical training needs. Several years back I began working with Gordon, and I have enjoyed a better understanding of functional exercise and its correlation to life's basic movements with associated strength, balance, and flexibility prioritization. Ironically, my cardio capabilities have also improved through this paradigm shift."

— Robert Brunswick,
CEO Buchannan Street Partners

"The best part of being a 73-year-old senior is being strong and looking young! Intelligently designed exercise programs coupled with a healthy diet and high-quality supplements have created stability and strength for my everyday activities. I strongly recommend the DFI personal training program for functional fitness because it works for everyone—especially seniors!"

—John Eagle,
Laguna Beach, CA

"I am a Blair Cervical Chiropractor who's been in practice for over twenty years. When my patients are seeing Gordon Duffy while under my care, they hold their adjustments longer and achieve better results from our treatments. I feel the Duffy Fitness Institute provides a very thorough evaluation, resulting in a customized exercise regimen that improves posture, performance, and health."

— Alfred W. Tomp, DC,
Rancho Santa Margarita, CA

7 EXERCISE MYTHS THAT ARE KILLING AMERICANS

7 Exercise Myths That Are Killing Americans:
The Ageless Truths That Will Keep You Fit, Functional and Fabulous for a Lifetime

ISBN: 978-0-9889362-0-1

Published by The Functional Fitness Institute

Book design by Stacey Aaronson,
www.creative-collaborations.com

The opinions expressed by the author are not necessarily those of The Functional Fitness Institute. This book is designed to provide accurate and authoritative information with regard to the subject matter covered. This information is given with the understanding that neither the author nor The Functional Fitness Institute is engaged in rendering legal, professional advice. Since the details of your situation are fact dependent, you should additionally seek the services of a competent professional.

MEDICAL ADVICE DISCLAIMER

THE AUTHOR PROVIDES THE BOOK IN ITS ENTIRETY, INCLUDING ITS CONTENT, SERVICES AND DATA (collectively, "Information") CONTAINED THEREIN, AND ONLY FOR THE PURPOSES OF INFORMATION. NO MEDICAL ADVICE IS PROVIDED IN THIS BOOK, AND THE INFORMATION SHOULD NOT BE USED OR UNDERSTOOD TO BE MEDICAL ADVICE. No aspect of use of the book constitutes a patient-physician relationship between you and the Author. This includes use of, reading the book, accessing and/or browsing the website, and/or providing any information to the Author. Nothing contained in the book is intended to take the place of or substitute for the services of a licensed, trained physician or health professional licensed in your state. Nothing in this book or on the website should be relied upon for making personal health decisions. A physician licensed in your state should be used for advice and consultation in all matters relating to your health. By use of this book and its website, you agree that you shall not make any health or medical-related decision based in whole or in part on anything contained in the book or on the website.

EXERCISE 7 MYTHS

THAT ARE

KILLING

AMERICANS

THE AGELESS TRUTHS THAT WILL KEEP YOU
FIT, FUNCTIONAL AND FABULOUS
FOR A LIFETIME

GORDON DUFFY

FFI

THE FUNCTIONAL FITNESS INSTITUTE

This book is dedicated to all who have struggled with their health, physically and emotionally, and have found a method to enhance both.

I also dedicate this book to those who are still struggling to find answers, truly value their health, and want to functionally extend their life.

With sincere humility, I offer the real truth within the pages you hold in your hand.

TABLE OF CONTENTS

PREFACE

I know what you're thinking: *How can exercise kill us? Surely exercise in any form is a good thing; as long as I'm moving and increasing my heart rate, I must be healthier than a sedentary person, right?*

Actually, the answer to that is *no*. I believe that many of the fitness strategies currently advocated by so-called experts are seriously harming the health of our citizens. That's why I wrote this book, to debunk some of the most widely held myths—for example, that sit-ups will result in great abs and that aerobic exercise is good for you—and instead introduce you to the ageless truths that will get you on the road to optimum fitness and functionality for a lifetime.

Most Americans aren't healthy, but they haven't a clue how unfit they really are in their ability to cope with life's everyday challenges.

I'll give you an example. Assuming an individual is ambulatory, which option—when given more than one—does he or she usually take: the escalator/elevator or the stairs? You guessed it: the one that requires the least exertion. It likewise doesn't help that the automated choice is often more available while the stairs are frequently tucked away and/or considered an emergency exit. Even if we're motivated to use them, they're not always conveniently located (and may even set off an alarm!).

This is merely one illustration of how society has provided us with hindrances to better health. To our disadvantage, the goal of making things *easier* has rarely equated to making us *healthier*, but then that correlation has never been the focus. For the sake of our generation and those to follow, the time has clearly come for a change.

In part because of our misguided beliefs about fitness, our kids are going to be even unhealthier than we are, not to mention we place more focus on winning competitive sports than getting fit for life. Our children are training year-round in the same sport with no break, and repetitive stress is injuring them, sometimes badly. In part this is because their coaches—who are often amateurs—don't have the training to implement programs that avoid injuries, nor have they learned how to adjust exercises to the needs of different age groups and physiques.

I recently held a camp in Pasadena for twenty-one kids aged thirteen to fifteen, and all of them had knee problems when they came to me. Why? Because they hadn't undergone physical evaluations to ensure that they were in good enough condition to engage in the kinds of physical activities demanded of them. They also weren't given appropriate strength training, yet they were being asked to play like professional athletes at a very young age, in most cases with little supervision and poor diets.

By striving to be the "best," competitively speaking, we are compromising our long-term health and probably shortening athletic careers.

We also put a priority on looking good rather than building optimum health and fitness, and this misguided focus risks long-term damage to our physiques and to our psyches.

Instead of using exercise to help keep our brains operating at the highest levels, we're doing the opposite, compromising our mental agility. We're stressing our bodies and minds rather than improving their functionality.

To summarize:

- ❖ We are misled by myths about fitness and suffer from a lack of education about the right way to exercise.

- ❖ Our focus on short-term goals, such as weight loss and winning at sports, is not in our best interest for maintaining lifelong, optimum health.

- ❖ Because we don't have our physical imbalances evaluated, we are unable to design corrective exercises.

- ❖ Our diets are dominated by poor food choices, such as processed and fast foods, and a lack of education about the impact of so-called "healthy foods" such as soy.

Earlier in the century, believe it or not, we were moving —pun intended—in a fairly reasonable direction. Less sedentary and more physically challenging lifestyles meant that people were getting varied types of exercise, and food was relatively unprocessed.

However, in the fifties and sixties—driven by profit motives—the food, agriculture, and chemical industries began to spiral out of control, mass producing more and more fast food at low cost, as well as foods treated with a range of chemicals and hormones. This abundance made it easy and inexpensive for us to eat poorly, while modern conveniences—such as dishwashers—reduced the physical demands of keeping house.

We grew fatter and fatter.

Enter the fitness industry.

In the seventies, achieving fitness became increasingly popular as research physiologists documented the health risks of obesity and the links between exercise and weight loss. Well-known figures such as Jane Fonda and Arnold Schwarzenegger offered popular programs designed to "get you the body you've always wanted."

People were anxious to lose weight quickly, and aerobics and step-aerobics classes helped them achieve that goal—but only in the short term. Ultimately—as we now know—most people focused on this form of exercise suffer cycles of weight gain and loss, and they lose muscle, which is detrimental as muscle is the key to burning fat.

We were "sold" on aerobics and extreme bodybuilding the same way we were convinced that margarine was better for us than butter (it isn't, by the way; olive oil is by far the preferred option). In the same way, we were led to believe that the food pyramid represented healthy eating (more on this later).

As time went on, more and more programs focused on helping people whose primary concern was to lose excess weight, which wouldn't necessarily improve their health or result in a loss of body fat.

Fitness became big business. And, as with all big business, sales and marketing schemes promised that the same product or program would work for millions of people. This is rarely true when it comes to exercise. Each of us has different bodies, ages, and health histories.

One size does not fit all.

Not too many years ago, I ended up in a wheelchair because I didn't understand the best way for *me* to achieve my highest level of fitness. Instead I joined the crowd, following the misguided advice that has plagued our industry for decades.

Like most people, I ascribed to the seven exercise myths that are slowly killing Americans. But today, I'm happy to say, I've learned my lesson and am healthier than ever, both mentally and physically.

Ultimately I was one of the fortunate ones. During the course of my career, my situation took a turn reminiscent of anecdotes in a book called *Outliers: The Story of Success* by Malcolm Gladwell. The author tells of successful people, such as Bill Gates and Steve Jobs, who in retrospect were at the right spot at the right time in history to make the most of their talents. Sometimes it's plain luck, good timing, the presence of just the right mentor for your particular talent, or emerging technology that is perfectly suited to your aptitude, along with hard work.

Mostly these people are smart enough to seize on the opportunities before them and make the most of the confluence of several key factors, including timing, the right mentors, and emerging insights in the field. I like to think I am one of those people. Why?

In the seventies, I was one of the first "fitness gurus" to specialize in personal training. In the eighties, I studied with some of the best in the business to become a strength and conditioning specialist. I worked hard to become a highly respected exercise physiologist/kinesiologist, offering unique and controversial but effective techniques to achieve ageless health. I'll outline many of them in this book.

I've embraced every learning opportunity and have been fortunate to gravitate toward experts who not only apply scientific methods proven to work clinically in the field, but also possess the potential to change people's lives. I've witnessed top athletes, physicians, and everyday people benefit from these data-driven techniques. I've watched exercise fads come and go over the years, from the aerobics craze of the seventies to the Crossfit phenomenon of today. Each has its drawbacks for reasons deeply rooted in our evolution as a species.

I have, in fact, tried most of these fad programs, and some of them were so hard on my body that I injured myself. You don't have to go through that same learning curve. I've been your guinea pig, and I can help you avoid the biggest pitfalls.

During my forty years in the industry, learning from my mistakes and using scientifically based research, I have structured a logical and workable approach to fitness, one that may reduce the symptoms of many illnesses. Some of these methods are going to seem counterintuitive to you, but that's only because of the vast amount of misinformation that has been drummed into us as a society over the years.

How do we know our approach to fitness has been misguided? Look around you. The truth is that the world population faces serious health deficiencies that are reaching epidemic proportions. Our children are reaching puberty faster than the generations preceding them, and diseases such as diabetes have proliferated despite our technological advancements.

Many experts agree that healthcare expenditures could be reduced by two-thirds if we took care of ourselves the way we should, and doing so isn't that difficult. The investment you need to make in order to stay healthy—a daily average of ten percent of your time—is far less burdensome than dealing with preventable illnesses.

I truly care about your health. I want you to live at the highest possible level of function so that you can enjoy a long and productive life. I feel driven to share the revolutionary anti-aging techniques that have been life changing for me and for my clients.

I hope that by pointing out the absurdity of some of the things we're doing and by educating about better ways to stay fit and functional, people will begin to lead healthier lives.

The generalization about Americans—and there's a lot of truth to this—is that we want everything to be fast. We want to see results *now*. We opt for pills that make us feel better, but we've forgotten what it's like to feel good in the first place.

Our information about health is one long, drug-company-sponsored infomercial, much of it with no real scientific basis in facts. Marketers are making huge profits, but the overall population isn't getting any healthier.

For example, depression is one of the top illnesses in the world right now. Do you know how we treat it? With medication. Yet what are some of the common side effects of antidepressants?

❖ Anxiety

❖ Agitation

❖ Decreased sex drive

❖ Increased depression

❖ Increased risk of suicide

Depressing, indeed. What's more, another pill is often prescribed to counteract the side effects of the first one. Interestingly, the additional pills are frequently from the same company that sold you the antidepressants. Further mixed messages exist concerning nutrition, and I will address these in the coming chapters.

I believe my colleagues and I possess key insights into how to keep a body in motion for a lifetime. By combining these insights with science-based techniques, we have a much better understanding of how exercise relates to fitness, overall health, and longevity—and how that can benefit us as individuals and as a nation.

What we recommend is a *functional* approach to fitness. By functional, I mean a strengthening and conditioning method that focuses on the natural movements of the human body, rather than artificial or repetitive physical activities that are more likely to do harm than good. This approach can work for everyone, and the methodology has been proven over time to thwart disease, combat degeneration, and contribute to hormone balance.

From our country's perspective, an overwhelming percentage of our medical care is focused on treatment, not prevention—a key reason why our healthcare costs are so high.

The bottom line: We need to become properly educated to avoid a national health catastrophe. If you're reading this book looking for ageless truths about exercise that will improve your quality of life, increase longevity, and optimize functionality, you've come to the right place.

When Americans embrace the truth about fitness, forget the fads, and work together to make a healthier nation for ourselves and future generations, we will all benefit.

HOW MY
FITNESS PHILOSOPHY EVOLVED

Growing up in the Southern California town of Pasadena in the fifties and sixties, I didn't have a great-looking body, to say the least. I was tall, extremely thin, and at one point had to deal with a serious case of acne.

Tank tops became popular when I was in high school, but I refused to wear one because I felt ashamed of my body. Girls teased me because of my stick-like physique, and though I suffered inside, their insults helped motivate me. To this day, despite many compliments, I still have body-image issues, and you won't see me in a tank top anytime soon (not a good look for most men, in my opinion).

While I was embarrassed by my appearance, I became determined to improve myself on my own terms. Lucky for me, my father was a nutritional chef, so my family always ate good food—even though we weren't financially well off—and we were taught to appreciate a balanced life.

Growing up, I had a strong desire to learn as much as I could academically, and my above-average hand-eye coordination allowed sports to be a very influential part of my life. I was in Little League and also played basketball and football. I must have had borderline ADD, because I couldn't sit still; I always had to be on the move. Because of my stringy physique, and despite my moments of success in sports, I experienced an underlying sense of insecurity. I didn't believe I could compete with the better athletes.

ARMY LIFE

In the seventies, I was drafted for two years and was one of the last draftees to go through the process. Though I had been born in Canada, I was a patriot and believed in the United States, so off I went to boot camp. I decided I would use the opportunity to develop myself physically and mentally.

In three weeks of basic training, I put on fifteen pounds. What's more, the Army taught me leadership skills and how to take initiative. I learned that respecting people who were more experienced than I was and following their lead was a much smarter strategy than thinking I knew all the answers. At one point, eight hundred other men and I were told that when someone asks for your name, you answer with your rank and your last name.

After leaving that lecture, the first question I heard was, "What's your name?" I said, "Private Duffy." Apparently I was the only guy who listened because everyone else gave their first names. As a result, they gave me temporary sergeant stripes.

When I first got to the base in Germany, they'd just finished building a brand new gym. With my renewed confidence—and muscle mass—I tried out for the decathlon contest and was selected to be on the team. I won a prestigious NATO event, receiving an award and high praise from a general. I also participated in Golden Glove boxing in Europe, winning in three different categories. I played all kinds of sports in between field duties as well.

I made some truly great friends from across the world, people who were also athletes and gracious enough to share their experience and expertise. I was also fortunate to have a highly respected officer take me on as an assistant. His mentoring was invaluable.

By the time I left the military, I'd become confident not only in my physical strength—putting on fifty-eight pounds in total—but in my intellectual capabilities.

WORKING AND WORKING OUT

After returning from the service, I found a job at a women's gym. I was full to the brim with knowledge I'd gained in Europe, which gave me a head start over other trainers in the business.

I saw that women could benefit from strength training, despite the conventional wisdom that said they'd build ugly muscle. I saw what happened when people focused on weight loss and not fat loss—they got thinner, at least for a while, but they didn't gain strength. From the beginning, for that and other reasons you'll see later in the book, I was not a fan of aerobics.

When I heard that a world-renowned fitness trainer named Bill Pearl also worked in Pasadena, I joined his gym. A legend in his field, an awesome person, and a man of the highest integrity, I knew he was the ideal guy to be my main mentor. Pearl, a multiple winner of the Mr. Universe title as well as a phenomenal writer and teacher, was for me "the right person at the right time." I trained at his gym for almost three years, building knowledge and applying it to myself and others.

I learned a lot from Bill about the fitness business—how to train individuals as well as other trainers. I'd get up, bike to the gym, and work with Bill from 5:15 to 7:20 every morning. It was during this time that I gleaned the best of the best knowledge out there and began to customize my approach to fitness.

I also trained at Gold's Gym at the same time as Arnold Schwarzenegger. During the seventies and eighties, bodybuilding had become widely focused on looks along with posing. I realized that bodybuilding wasn't the only way —or the ideal way—to train to be an athlete and get healthy, and that many people attempting to create a "beautiful body" suffered serious negative side effects, such as bad posture and poor functional health. We now know that bodybuilding may, over time, actually decrease our ability to perform everyday activities, especially as we age. It simply makes sense to focus on functionality from the beginning, enabling us to perform everyday activities efficiently, no matter what our age.

The owner of the women's gym where I worked decided that the gym should go coed, which was unique at the time. Business exploded, and I was teaching fitness classes in the evenings. After a while, I pretty much took over the running of the gym, almost without anyone—including myself—really noticing how much responsibility I had assumed. I was essentially working two jobs—sales and marketing—and training while earning my Masters in Sports degree with the International Sports Science Association (ISSA).

ISSA was founded by Dr. Frederick C. Hatfield, an intellect and the first person to squat over a thousand pounds competitively, and by Dr. Sal A. Arria, an expert in physiology. Bill Pearl and Paul Chek were on the ISSA Committee, which meant I was learning from the best powerlifters in the business, as well as soaking up the expertise of exercise physiologists who had done extensive clinical research. I reread all the relevant books and gathered information from the field, while Chek helped fine-tune my skills in writing up professional evaluations and training plans.

During that period, I also studied with and was certified by the Poliquin Institute. Paul Chek and Charles Poliquin are two of the best trainers in the world, and although their work is so sophisticated that it is sometimes hard for the layman to understand the logic behind their methods, they are proven to work and I've integrated them into my approach.

Working with the highest level of experts in the fitness field increased my desire to learn the truth beyond the myths. My search for the perfect fitness regime, adaptable for different individuals, began in earnest.

OVERKILL

During this time I participated in sports including boxing, basketball, football, and even team handball, which was relatively unknown at the time. The variety of experience I gained at work and play, along with my interactions with so many different personalities, hugely increased my knowledge base and honed my teaching skills.

I offered personal training before it was a common concept, with clients from the entertainment business to athletes at amateur and professional levels. Also, an acquaintance who worked at NBC introduced me to influential people in the television industry, which also helped me gain exposure.

In my failure to understand fitness myths, I was doing hundreds of sit-ups a day while training my clients, which I would later learn was a serious mistake. The repetitive exercises began to hurt my back. The importance of correct posture was neglected in those days, and I didn't realize I was doing too much forward-leaning exercise.

My subsequent injuries led to one of the epiphanies that would help shape my fitness philosophy. However, because my work schedule was so intense at the time, I continued to ignore what my body was telling me: that I was working too hard. I got sick a few times and ended up with a serious kidney disorder that put me down for nearly a year and a half. While recovering, I studied nutrition with the help of my father, who believed in a holistic approach. His advice about scientifically based nutrition was instrumental in getting my kidneys working efficiently again—and that, too, informed my approach to fitness.

During the early nineties, I made the same mistake again. I worked two jobs—fitness training and sales—and I became exhausted. But I was so fit overall and looked so good that the doctors didn't take me seriously. One day I finally broke down completely. I was diagnosed with an obstinate case of acute mononucleosis.

Frustrated is a nice way of saying it.

I was angry with myself, but I turned my breakdown into a learning opportunity. With the approval of my mentors and based on my research, I started doing immune IV drips, which put high levels of Vitamin C directly into my bloodstream. I got well faster than the doctors anticipated. I had my body and kidneys back, and I was feeling great.

Four or five years later, still in the nineties, I opened my fitness institute in Laguna Beach. And then my back gave out and I broke down again. Because of my debilitating back injury, I thought my business was doomed. This former athlete and personal trainer couldn't walk. I was now in a wheelchair.

I thought I knew what I was doing, that I was focusing on the right things to stay healthy, but still I went down. I feared I was going to end up with debilitating back pain for the rest of my life. I didn't think I was going to be able to teach or train—my real love—or have any kind of normal life. I hit an emotional, physical, and intellectual wall. My identity was gone. Luckily, I had true-blue friends who were there for me.

I underwent surgery, which was originally going to be major, but ended up being (relatively) minor—not that any back surgery is ever easy—and during rehabilitation I entered the CHEK Institute, run by Paul Chek, who had already played a big role in influencing my thinking about smart approaches to good health. Chek is an international expert on corrective and high-performance exercise kinesiology who works with people recovering from injuries, teaching them how to move without exacerbating the problem.

Full rehabilitation took me nearly three arduous years.

About the same time, my father passed away and I helped care for my mother, who, then in her nineties, lived in a convalescent home. Despite the excellent outcome of my surgery, there were nights I had to sleep on the floor in my mother's room, which wasn't the best strategy for full rehabilitation. I had a hard time standing and walking and was reduced to crawling around on the floor of her room. Some help I was.

While caring for my mother, I caught a brain virus, which I believe was primarily from the copper poisoning of the pipes at the convalescent home. I felt like Job in the Old Testament. *How many major setbacks can one person take?* I wondered. I told myself there had to be a purpose behind it all, and I began to research homeopathic remedies and speak to experts all over the world.

On top of the brain virus, the mononucleosis apparently had never completely left me, and I felt lethargic much of the time. Once again I took a regimen of immune drips with Vitamin C, made a full recovery, and restarted my business yet again. I humbly resolved to manage my life in an entirely different manner.

Shortly after I recovered from the brain virus, my brother passed away. Then my mother, who had been strict but very loving, died. I wondered if the obstacles of life were always going to keep me from moving on, but I slowly put myself back together emotionally.

During that time I rebuilt my business, recovered from surgery, and studied with Paul Chek, and I began to understand where I had gone wrong in my fitness philosophy and started practicing exercise techniques that resulted in my full recovery.

FIT AGAIN

When I recovered my fitness, I knew that my destiny was to share what I'd learned and help Americans become and stay healthy. In the long run, my health challenges have made me a better teacher. I became passionate about sharing with people what I had learned over the years and debunking the myths that had debilitated me.

Finally, in 2006, I opened up Duffy Fitness in Irvine, California. Since then, I've combined the most respected research and scientifically backed protocols into a logical and comprehensive philosophy of fitness. (I've mentioned several people whose contributions to my program have been invaluable; I'd like to also give a shout-out to Dawn Van Ness, who always believed in the value of my methodologies.)

With the Duffy Fitness system—in addition to making hundreds of people leaner, stronger, and healthier—I have successfully rehabilitated hundreds of clients from back injuries and illnesses over the last ten years.

Our programs work.

I also train healthy people to maintain their fitness and improve their functionality as they age. We may not be able to stop the clock, but we can certainly increase the quality of our lives. All of my clients and friends who have incorporated my protocols are vibrant, living proof of this methodology.

As you've seen, I've had more than my share of physical setbacks. I've endured a serious spinal injury; I've experienced a couple of quirky illnesses. I know what it feels like to lose function. It's awful. Without the health problems and neurological issues caused by stress and poor exercise, we'd all be a lot happier.

NUTRITION THAT MAKES SENSE

As with exercise, I want to see people eating right, too. The benefits are greater than simply getting in better physical and mental shape.

A recent study featured an experiment at a maximum-security prison for men, where the prisoners were fed organic food for ninety days. The rates of violence decreased substantially (the results are detailed at: www.ox.ac.uk/media/news-stories/2008/080129.html). Imagine what organic eating can do for everyone.

The cascading results of better nutrition and exercise affect not only you and your family, but society as well. We know that eating the right foods produces healthy minds and bodies that can function harmoniously. It's not hard to see that eating poorly can produce conflict, not only within the mind and body, but also among individuals and eventually within society. And we know that most of us are making poor food choices. How healthy we are as a civilization is tied to our nutritional options.

ANTI-AGING IS SIMPLY SCIENTIFIC

Contrary to what you may have come to believe, you *can* alter the biological clock once you understand the truth about anti-aging protocols and how they synergistically and scientifically work together. Good choices can actually alter genes; you don't have to believe you've been dealt a bad hand—I'm a perfect example.

The key to longevity is to take an intelligent, strategic, and serious look at health goals and find smart, foolproof answers. For example, why is the number one New Year's resolution for eighty percent of the American population always weight loss? Statistically, by Valentine's Day, that resolution is broken because what people engage in as a quick fix doesn't work. *Weight* loss is the wrong mindset; it's *fat* loss that is necessary. Following a trend isn't going to provide the know-how to optimize health goals and create a longer life; rather knowledge of how to balance hormones, enhance cellular healing, and decrease inflammation, oxidative stress, and damage from free radicals and toxins is what we need. I'm going to show you how.

Some of the most common anti-aging questions that inspired me to find truthful answers and share them with you are:

❖ How do Americans burn the fat we so desperately want to get rid of?

❖ What are the real keys to the fountain of youth?

❖ How do Americans maximize health with minimal time constraints?

❖ How do we work smarter, look younger, and feel fabulous?

While this book's emphasis is on which protocols NOT to use, I also offer advice on better approaches. By reading the following chapters, I want you to learn not only *how* to exercise (and eat) well, but to understand *why* certain exercises are better for you than others. We need to appreciate how muscle is built and its many functions, as well as the importance of posture, why exercise has such a strong effect on neurological function, and how exercise can keep you looking and feeling younger.

I want to be able to look back on my life and say, "I had an impact on making people healthier in this country."

With your help, we can do it together.

MYTH 1

AEROBIC EXERCISE IS THE BEST WAY TO LOSE FAT AND GET FIT

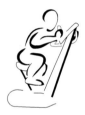

TRUTH:

Fat loss plateaus within weeks,
and aerobic exercise causes some negative health effects.

✗ **Aerobic Exercise and Survival Mode:**
Boom and bust weight cycles

✗ **The Aerobic Exercise Physique:**
It's not pretty

✗ **The Aerobic Heart:**
Heart efficiency will not prevent heart problems

According to the Centers for Disease Control (CDC),[1] the latest statistics show that sixty-eight percent of Americans are overweight or obese. Does that sixty-eight percent consist of people who never exercise or do aerobics? No. Plenty of those people have danced to hours of videotapes or run marathons. What's gone wrong?

---

[1] Cynthia L. Ogden, PhD, and Margaret D. Carroll, MSPH, Division of Health and Nutrition Examination Survey, *Prevalence of Overweight, Obesity, and Extreme Obesity Among Adults: United States, Trends 1960–1962 through 2007–2008*, Washington, DC: Government Printing Office, 2010.

Since the sixties delivered the start of the running craze and the seventies saw Americans embrace aerobics, we have been told that as long as we move a great deal in a short period of time, we'll become healthy, lose weight, and add muscle. But as a nation we're only getting fatter and unhealthier. Why?

Unfortunately, many people touting the benefits of repetitive aerobic exercise were not certified or academically qualified to make any such recommendations. It was as though we invested in bad stock, one that had an immediate positive impact—people lost weight in the short term—but over time they didn't make long-term health gains, as I'll explain in this chapter.

We see the mantra repeated over and over: If you want to lose weight and improve your health, there's no better way than to do it aerobically!

Aerobic exercise gets rid of your muscles as fast as it gets rid of fat. But muscle burns fat, so losing muscle is not a good strategy for long-term weight loss.

Despite the now-obvious fact that aerobic exercise isn't effective, many people still tout its benefits. Several Hollywood celebrities have become fitness gurus, and seeing their fabulous figures persuades many people that repetitive exercise is the way to go. Trouble is, most of them looked good before they started promoting their methods. The routines didn't give them their gorgeous bodies; their phenomenal genes did. Yet people continue to think they can achieve figures like celebrities if they follow their advice. And from a marketing perspective, the alternatives to aerobics are so far under the radar that nobody knows about them.

People think, *I'm putting on weight, so I better start running and doing sit-ups*, because that's what we see on TV. I thought the same for a long time. I'd say, "Oh boy, I'd better get in shape; I should start running," and then I would run too far and injure myself.

Promoters of aerobic exercise will tell you it's the best way to:

❖ Stay off the yo-yo dieting cycle

❖ Lose a lot of weight

❖ Gain a decent amount of muscle

❖ Start a fitness program for the first time

❖ Avoid heart problems

❖ Avoid a bad back or bad knees

❖ Reduce stress in your life

People selling aerobics classes often say that all you have to do to be fit is get moving; and the more you get moving, the healthier you'll be; and as long as you're moving, it doesn't matter what kind of physique you have.

It turns out that fitness is a bit more complex. There's an aerobic and anaerobic side to most types of athletic activity, but to emphasize the aerobic side only will not accomplish weight-loss goals. Ninety-nine percent of the time, this approach fails.

Aerobic training tends to cause weight cycling in people who don't do it consistently, which contributes to hormonal imbalances and long-term muscle loss rather than fat loss. On top of that, unlike other types of training, aerobic training will not:

❖ Improve brain function

❖ Support your skeletal system, posture, or prevent injury

❖ Increase your bone density

Bottom line: Aerobic exercise will not make you more functional. Yes, you do need to get moving, but not in a way that will do more harm than good. Let me explain.

EXERCISE AND SURVIVAL MODE

In nature, animals mostly operate anaerobically, which means they go from a start to a stop pretty explosively—to hunt and to escape from danger—but seldom run for miles without stopping, or repeat similar actions in a short period of time.

If you look at the human animal and examine the different types of sports that have evolved over time, almost every single one is based on anaerobic exercise that incorporates explosive starting and stopping: soccer, baseball, basketball, rugby, football, and tennis, for example. Even golf isn't based on endurance but on explosive swing speed broken by periods of watchfulness and highly focused attention. Sports evolved to help us hone our ability to survive in a hostile world.

So you can see that aerobic exercise isn't our bodies' natural choice. In fact, it's so far from what our bodies see as normal that after about six weeks of performing any given type of aerobic exercise, they go into survival mode, the same way as if we were starving. Parts of your body and mind actually shut down.

Dancing with a pair of minuscule weights may get your heart rate up, and you might burn some fat (along with muscle), but it's not going to help you live longer, nor will it help your posture. And after six weeks, you're not going to see a lot of weight loss either, because the body says: "Okay, I've adapted to this survival challenge you've thrown at me, and now I can afford to add some fat cells again, which I know you're going to need because I've learned now that our life is always at stake."

When your body goes into survival mode:

❖ First, it does whatever it takes to get you through the situation (a phase where you lose weight).

❖ Second, it adapts (a phase where you stop losing weight).

❖ Finally it adds more fat, because fat is what helps you survive when you're in survival mode (a phase where you gain weight, doing the same amount of exercise). The fat returns, because you have worked extremely hard at convincing your body that you need to conserve it.

If you want to consistently lose weight, don't put your body in survival mode; it's just an invitation for it to add fat reserves as soon as possible.

THE ANTI-AGING TRUTH ABOUT AEROBICS

Aerobic training, according to recent studies, isn't an effective anti-aging exercise strategy for balancing hormones, losing fat, or staying slim. *But aerobics has been around for awhile now*, you're probably thinking, *and some of my friends have gotten good results*. Think again.

> **Oxidative Stress** | äk-sə-'dā-tiv 'stres
> noun
> occurs when the body produces more chemically-reactive molecules containing oxygen (or Reactive Oxygen Species [ROS]) than it can handle.

Cardio—or aerobic—fitness can actually accelerate the aging process. Very simply, when engaging in long, low-intensity exercise, you increase oxidative stress, which ages you and lowers growth hormone production and testosterone. Over time, the oxidative stress can raise cortisol levels and lead to fat *storage* instead of fat *burning*, creating inflammation.[2] Systemic or chronic inflammation has a domino effect that can seriously undermine your health. What's more, when you keep your heart rate in the fat-burning zone during aerobic activity for one hour, you can burn fat during that time; however, studies have proven that you can also burn muscle for the next twenty-four to thirty-six hours. The opposite is true for exercise that increases muscle, lowers cortisol production, and increases testosterone and growth hormones. A good strength-training or burst-training program will help to burn sugar and fat twenty-four to thirty-six hours after exercising.[3]

---

[2] "How to Counter the Many Negatives of Aerobic Training"
http://www.charlespoliquin.com/ArticlesMultimedia/Articles/Article/734/
How_to_Counter_The_Many_Negatives_of_Aerobic_Train.aspx

[3] Secret #4 of the 5 Secrets to Anti-Aging | Health Tips – Dr. Pompa
http://www.drpompa.com/Health-Tips/burst-training-best-exercise-for-longevity.html

THE AEROBICS PHYSIQUE

If you're doing aerobic exercise in order to look good, keep in mind—as I mentioned—that the people who are doing a lot of aerobic exercise and looking good doing it, such as Jane Fonda, already looked good before they started.

Bottom line, if you do a lot of aerobics, you may be able to get a physique like Richard Simmons, but probably not Jamie Lee Curtis's. Her genes are on her side.

Think of the top ten most attractive people in the world. With all due respect, I bet Richard Simmons isn't on that list. Sadly, many people who swear by aerobics aren't the picture of health. Their skin sags because they've lost muscle mass along with body fat. Among people who have been doing aerobics and dieting rigorously for years, you'll even see a few who look like victims of starvation.

Many of the women who did Richard Simmons' program lost plenty of weight. I knew several who lost close to two hundred pounds or more, at least in the short term. However, their arms tended to be flabby, indicating that they hadn't lost as much body fat as you might imagine. And if the weight they lost wasn't a hundred percent fat, where was the rest of that weight coming from? Muscle.

The latest studies have shown that muscle cells burn three times as many calories as fat cells. By losing muscle, you're increasing the chances that you'll rebound and gain the weight back, because you'll lower your metabolic rate and won't be burning the same amount of calories at the same rate as before.

LONG-DISTANCE RUNNING

We as a species are not genetically engineered to run long distance, and most people shouldn't, which is why most of my cardio exercise comes from weight training or sprints.

Running can be a good thing if you're training for a specific goal, are already in shape, and know how to do it. But running long distances will only serve to get average Americans where they want to be geographically, not physically.

I once saw two people trying to run who were each around a hundred pounds overweight. The guy leaned forward, looking at his feet, and the woman's knees were at awkward angles. They ran around the block a couple of times, probably trying to lose weight, not training for a serious event.

Unfortunately, running is not a logical way for such people to accomplish their goals of losing weight and getting healthy.

People who choose to run must have a physical assessment done to ensure their bodies are fit enough to take on the challenge, whether they are marathoners, sprinters, or weekend warriors.

One fifty-five-year-old client of mine was very statuesque and attractive when I first evaluated her. She was in love with running and came to me with a hip problem. Daily, she ran at least five or six miles; she also ran frequently on the treadmill. But regardless of her cardiovascular fitness, her hip problems persisted. I told her we were going to have to change how she exercised, because obviously something she was doing wasn't working in her favor.

I only worked with her for a short time before she stopped coming to the gym, but two years later she returned. Two things had changed. One, she hadn't done the weight training I had recommended; and two, she'd become a vegetarian. Now she looked anorexic; she had dropped probably seventy pounds. I could see every bone in her back, every angle of the joints in her shoulder. Her hair was falling out because she wasn't getting enough protein or fat, yet when I talked to her about her fitness strategies, she said, "It's going great! My hips don't hurt. I've lost so much weight that the pressure on them is better. I want to add some strength training to my program, but I still want to be able to run five or six miles a day."

She thought she looked good. Her physique was typical of people who do a lot of long-distance running: stringy, with more than a hint of bone. She was conforming to the notion that the archetypal healthy person is a stick-thin, vegetarian marathoner, but in actuality, truly attractive people brim with vitality.

Despite the misconceptions, I understand the lure of running. It produces a lot of endorphins, which are literally the body's own morphine (the word *endorphin* is a contraction of "endogenous morphine"). My client was addicted, not to alcohol or prescription drugs, but to running.

If you combine consistent aerobic exercise with starving yourself, you'll get the physique of a marathoner. Is that the figure you really want?

People who become addicted to endorphin highs may be obsessive-compulsive, which means they do more and more aerobic exercise, compounding their health problems. On the other hand, a lot of people who run quit after a short period of time because they injure themselves. Further, in my opinion, people who have heart problems shouldn't be running at all. This is especially important to keep in mind for people who are over fifty. There's nothing wrong with running a marathon or going on a long bike ride once in a while, but it's not going to build up the physical and mental strength you need as you get older.

Runners frequently end up with knee, back, and neck problems. For years I've worked with these so-called "in-shape" clients who tend to pay little attention to the structure, stability, and alignment of their bodies. Yes, they can run far and are often slim, but they injure themselves doing something as simple as lifting a box from a shelf or playing a game of golf. Also, unbeknownst to most people, it's difficult to add muscle by running. When you do steady aerobic, cardiovascular work, your muscles are acutely compromised.

Marathon runners deserve accolades, because what they do can be impressive in setting and accomplishing tough physical goals. But most of us aren't built to be marathon runners. The men who excel are usually around five foot nine and weigh approximately one hundred and ten pounds with twig-like upper arms. East African men are particularly successful at this sport, but these marathoners have adapted their bodies over generations, beginning to run not long after they learn to walk. For them, it's a national sport.

In order for most of us to get into that shape, we'd have to destroy a lot of muscle along with the fat, and if we're carrying extra weight (or don't have a perfectly aligned structure), we're going to hurt ourselves in the process. Women who lose a great deal of weight too quickly put their hearts in danger, too, which we'll explore further in Myth 2.

THE AEROBIC HEART

Most people think that aerobic activity makes your heart *efficient*, but that's not the same as making your heart *stronger*. In order to strengthen your heart, you need to train anaerobically.

So what does aerobic activity do for you? Let's think of your heart as a pump, which it is. In order to make your heart more efficient, you must train it to do the same things over and over again: to empty itself out and take on more fluid. The more often you do this, the more your heart develops a structure that helps it pump fluid faster and more efficiently.

For example, imagine running one mile with a certain amount of effort; then running two miles with more or less the same effort, and so on. You become more efficient at eating up those miles. But you're not increasing the intensity, only the reps, so your heart isn't getting stronger, only better adapted to running long distances. Your endurance increases, but not your ability to handle stress. In fact, aerobic training plateaus after eight weeks at most; anything else is counterproductive.

If your goal is to get stronger, forget aerobics. In the long term, it will actually make you slower and weaker.

Why? In part because you're placing your focus on too few muscles instead of strengthening your overall functionality.

Consider five hundred reps of a one-pound weight. This method is not going to help you lift a five-pound weight, or a fifty-pound weight, or even a five-hundred-pound weight. The marathon runner or aerobics fanatic can keep moving all day long, but that won't mean that he or she will be able to lift a barbell—or his or her kids—any more easily. People like to run because it's cheap and easy to get started, but it is by no means the best way to lose weight or gain fitness; it's just too easy to injure yourself.

Let's take the example of people within their normal weight range and give them 25-45 pound weights in a backpack to carry while they're running. If you try to run a long distance at any amount of speed with extra weight on you, you aren't going to feel good. You may lose weight at first, but not only do you risk injury, you're going to lose muscle tissue along with the fat, and your metabolic rate will go down once you stop running. Likewise, long-distance running doesn't burn much fat.

Think about it. Who has less fat, a sprinter or a marathoner? It's pretty obvious who has more muscle—the sprinter—but the sprinters have less body fat despite the fact they do almost zero continuous aerobic work. They have higher-intensity workouts, which drive a higher maximum heart rate and burn more calories per minute. Of course, the athletes who tamper with their bodies using drugs don't have that same life expectancy, but the people who train from a clean standpoint naturally have much stronger hearts.

> Sprinters and weight trainers who train correctly have a tendency to live a very long time.

With a strong heart, when you get into a stressful situation—either an everyday challenge or a situation where you need to push yourself physically—you're going to be able to handle it, because your heart is strong enough to keep up. Aerobics, on the other hand, doesn't enhance functionality and, if overused, can cause serious harm.

MORE ON OXIDATIVE STRESS

Oxidation is a natural process that happens in your body when oxygen binds with other substances. In most cases, oxidation is good, but sometimes our bodies have a tendency to acquire too much oxygen.

ROS (Reactive Oxygen Species) easily combines with molecules such as amino acids, and this may prevent them from carrying out their normal functions. Too much aerobic—or air-carrying—exercise causes the worst amount of oxidative stress.

Long-distance training builds oxidative stress, which research suggests can be aging at a cellular level. It also impacts the balance of hormones in your body, causing premature aging and difficulty in achieving weight loss. Anti-aging strategies are really quite simple: keep cells healthy and avoid inflammation.

While oxygen is vital for life, too much can cause damage to cells, DNA, enzymes, and more. Some experts believe that as an immediate effect of oxidation, doing too much aerobic exercise drops your IQ by about fifty percent. Research findings agree that you can't think clearly until your body clears out the excess ROS.

Free radicals are a direct result of ROS caused by oxidation. They occur when oxygen binds with molecules it shouldn't, leaving behind molecules with extra or missing parts, and an electrical charge (which acts like static electricity, making them "stick" to other molecules). This chain reaction leads to tissue damage and dysfunction.

Normally the body can neutralize free radicals in one of two ways: certain enzyme chains take up the free radicals for use, or antioxidants bind with the free radicals and stop the chain reaction from happening. When you don't have enough antioxidants in your body to neutralize the free radicals, your metabolism begins to run slower and less efficiently. Carrying around too many free radicals may make you age more quickly, as your cells are unable to repair all the damage being caused.

The problem with aerobic activity is that it is meant to increase the amount of oxygen in your body. More oxygen leads to more free radicals, which leads to more damage, and damaging your body obviously isn't going to make you look good.

ADRENAL STRESS

Another downside of aerobic training is that it promotes adrenal stress, which can make you fatter and cause other health problems. Your adrenal glands, located just above your kidneys, handle your body's response to stress via hormones like cortisol, a steroid that increases blood sugar and suppresses the immune system in order to boost your energy for handling an immediate challenge. Adrenal glands also produce adrenaline, which increases your heart rate, dilates your air passages, and more. These hormones and others are part of your fight-or-flight reaction to emergencies, but they can also be triggered by all kinds of stress, from exercise to job pressure to not getting enough sleep.

When you do too much continuous aerobic exercise, your adrenal glands are stressed constantly, which upsets the delicate balance between pumping up the body to respond to an emergency and leaving the body in maintenance mode. With high levels of stress, your immune system is always

"Normal functioning in adrenal glands secrete minute-by-minute yet precise balance amounts of steroid hormones."

——Dr. James Wilson, author of Adrenal Fatigue: The 21st Century Stress Syndrome

suppressed and you'll get sick more frequently. You may also have too much glucose in the bloodstream, as a stressful event may put your body into a fight-or-flight reaction, causing an immediate surge in blood sugar to give you the fuel you need to react to a threatening situation. When in this mode, you will constantly receive too much oxygen and may experience symptoms associated with adrenal fatigue such as:

- ❖ Tiredness
- ❖ Fearfulness
- ❖ Allergies
- ❖ Frequent influenza
- ❖ Arthritis
- ❖ Anxiety

- ❖ Depression
- ❖ Reduced memory function
- ❖ Difficulty in concentrating
- ❖ Insomnia
- ❖ The inability to lose weight after extensive efforts

Cortisol also affects the body's ability to tell whether you've had enough to eat. Increased cortisol levels lead to increased hunger as your body tries to store up enough energy——in the form of fat——to deal with the next crisis.

In our modern lives, we already go through a lot of stress. Adding more by doing continuous aerobic training is going to increase body fat and make it harder to reach your weight-loss goals.

EXERCISE-INDUCED CASTRATION

Not only is aerobic exercise making you look worse, but it's holding you back from optimal sexual health. When you're stressed, your sex drive is lessened because the adrenal glands also produce the sex hormones testosterone, progesterone, and estrogen. Your body basically says, "Sex is not the priority; survival is" and stops producing normal levels of sex hormones. Too much aerobic exercise can stress your body to the point where you don't want to have sex.

As Coach Poliquin notes, "Continuous aerobic work is basically exercise-induced castration."

PHYSICAL INJURIES

Because people are different and have varied lifestyles and capabilities, it's just not possible to train a million people using the exact same protocol. Some are understandably more genetically predisposed to succeed with one program than another.

Step aerobics is probably the worst form of exercise people could choose. Alternately placing one foot up and the other down puts stress on your hip joints. When you bring both feet up on top of the platform, you take stress briefly off the hip joint, but do it over and over and it becomes a repetitive stress. The period of time that the hip joint spends under tension isn't long enough to develop the muscle; the step up, step down motion actually doesn't build muscle at all. It's simply stressing the joint again and again.

Jane Fonda is famous for her step-aerobics workouts, but she had to have a hip replacement in June 2005 because she had damaged the joint so badly as a result. She's a beautiful lady with a lovely figure, but I think if she had understood the negative impact of aerobics and the damage it can do to joints, she wouldn't have taught it. But because she wasn't educated about the potential for injuries, she unwittingly caused a lot of harm to people who followed her program.

WHY AEROBICS IS NEVERTHELESS STILL POPULAR

It's easy to get caught up in a sense that you've never lost enough weight, or that you're never trim enough. But a lack of muscle isn't attractive, whether you're losing a lot of weight or just trimming off those last few ounces. It's better to have reserves of muscle to support you and keep you looking svelte, instead of portraying the picture of a famine victim.

Aerobic exercise can be good for the short term, but only if you're starting out with an extreme weight problem and follow a low-impact program that doesn't cause repetitive stress on the joints. There's value in simply getting people to move when they're first starting out with exercise;

however, investing in aerobic activity is again like investing in bad stock that performs well over a six-week period—because that's about all you get with any aerobic activity before your body adapts—but after that loses value.

What you need to invest in for the long term is muscle, but you must do so by being smart in your workout to avoid injury. Six-pack abs and other muscle imbalances defeat anti-aging goals. Our programs build muscle for functionality and longevity, bringing balance to your body's structure, alignment, and stability, stimulating the right mix of hormones for optimal lifetime health.

CRITICAL TAKEAWAY

FOCUS ON REDUCING BODY FAT RATHER THAN LOSING POUNDS AS AN OVERALL WEIGHT-LOSS STRATEGY.

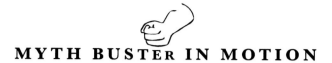

MYTH BUSTER IN MOTION

The best way to lose fat, enhance metabolic rate for stable, long-term changes, and improve muscle tone is through **high-intensity interval training** and **strength-training** protocols.

High-intensity training is done in short periods of time with repetitions and rest periods.

- ❖ Perform exercises for two minutes at a high intensity.
- ❖ Rest for 60-90 seconds (depending on the shape you are in to bring the heart rate back down to a normal rate).
- ❖ Repeat that exercise for another two minutes; rest for 60-90 seconds.
- ❖ Do this for 15-20 minutes to properly increase heart rate for maximum impact.

Strength training builds muscle, burns fat, lowers cortisol and inflammation, and provides long-term anti-aging health results. A few suggestions are:

- ❖ Squats
- ❖ Dead lifts
- ❖ Lunges
- ❖ Cable Pulls
- ❖ Wall Push-Ups
- ❖ Lateral Ball Rolls

Utilize this regimen three days a week to optimize fat loss.

For more information on these specific exercises, visit:
www.ageless-human.com

MYTH 2

EXERCISE IS ONLY FOR THE BODY

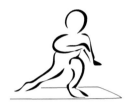

TRUTH:

The main purpose of exercise is to improve overall functioning, including mental acuity.

Strength Training:
Positive physical and mental impact

Effects of Aging:
Caring for your synapses

Managing Diabetes:
Appropriate diet and exercise is key

Exercising the right way is the key to staying mentally, as well as physically, healthy and fit. As we get older, we—or most of us!—recognize that looks are not as important as keeping our bodies and brains working well. And it's not a trade-off. You can have both a great appearance and optimum functionality.

Your brain is the ultimate center of your body; it's the organ that dictates everything that happens inside you, facilitating messages throughout your body via your nervous system.

Many of our clients are seventy and older, and they enjoy great physical function and a positive mindset. Using our fitness programs, they have rebuilt their "mental muscles" as much as their physical ones, keeping them sharp and aware. Some run twenty-yard wind sprints—running back and forth over twenty yards, as fast as they can—among other exercises. One seventy-seven-year-old runs faster than most people I know.

Here's the caveat: not all types of exercise will rebuild your mental muscles for you. You may look good but not be functioning at the highest levels.

As we've seen, too much aerobic exercise reduces brain and physical function through oxidative stress. Also, aerobics is repetitive—mindlessly so—and gets your brain into certain habits of doing the same thing over and over, rather than training it to deal with differing challenges. Because there are no major changes to most aerobics programs, the brain begins to flatline.

Similar to running for extended periods of time, aerobic activity causes your metabolism to dip because your body doesn't know how much it's going to be called on to do and therefore preserves its resources. Your brain likewise goes on autopilot. Ask anyone who's been stranded in the wilderness for an extended period of time—they start losing brain function, because the brain actually slows down so it can survive.

Another example of wrong-headed exercises (to coin a phrase) in the opinion of experts is jumping jacks. These actually reverse your brain function because they don't conform to natural human movement, meaning they're not an appropriate movement pattern from a kinesiological point of view.

Kinesiology | kə-ˌnē-sē-ˈä-lə-jē
noun
(also known as Kinetics)
the scientific study of human movement.

Imagine you're an octopus: It takes a lot of brain function to organize eight limbs. You may think, *How hard could it be?* But try walking with a pair of crutches for the first time, and you'll realize how difficult it is to coordinate four legs. Likewise, your brain is calculating some really complex physics when you coordinate activities among a range of muscles.

An octopus is, in fact, one of the most intelligent of non-mammalian species. They're known for their ability to escape confinement and make raids on fish three tanks over. Their brains get a workout from organizing eight limbs that don't do the same repetitive things, but rather deal with all kinds of obstacles and challenges, from navigating tricky tidal currents to finding food. This is what I mean by increasing functionality: *enhancing your ability to meet the mental and physical demands that everyday life places on you.*

> Your muscles may be able to perform all kinds of amazing feats, but if you're not programming your brain to utilize them effectively in the real world, you're not achieving much.

Yes, perhaps you can move your biceps up and down longer than your friends, or jog in place for hours, or do record numbers of jumping jacks, but your mind isn't any sharper. If anything, it has probably gone into a coma of sorts, dulled by repetitive action.

Repetitive exercise doesn't improve your ability to solve physical or mental problems—you've only forged neural pathways necessary to lift weights or stair-step. Back and forth, up and down: that's the only movement you've taught your brain to handle.

Your nervous system is a chain of command: brain to nerves, nerves to muscles. The more you practice giving appropriate, life-logical commands, the better your muscles, nerves, and brain will perform.

Exercise can vastly improve how well you think and how effectively you function in the world. The benefits of exercising properly can be shockingly simple and highly effective.

For example, one Duffy Fitness client is a well-known financial manager. When he came to us, he could barely walk forward, and he couldn't walk backward at all. He'd either fall or freeze, trying to figure out how to make his body move the way he wanted. He was also having great difficulty falling asleep. The man was a dysfunctional mess. All his life he had been a bookworm and when he wasn't in his office, he loved to work in libraries studying finance. At sixty-five years of age, he didn't play sports or do anything that physically stimulated his brain.

I recommended an exercise we call cross-crawling, which is a way to reprogram the nervous system and remind the brain how to get all our systems working together effectively. Simple as it sounds, this approach had terrific results. After utilizing it for about a year, he was able to walk forward and backward with ease and do a one-legged squat without holding onto anything. He says his workload has tripled, yet he's able to do more in less time because his mental acuity has increased. Exercise based on kinetics may sometimes require patience but has excellent results.

Maybe you're not in a situation where you need to see that kind of improvement, but everyone has physical and mental functionality to maintain as they age, and most would agree that functionality should take priority over appearance.

STRENGTH TRAINING

What exercises make the most sense to increase physical and mental health? The answer is strength training, focused on natural human movement.

First, strength training has immense physical impact. Muscle burns fat—I can't emphasize that enough—so fat loss is also a benefit of strength training. For some reason, as we were doing countless crunches and hundreds of hours of aerobics, strength was never emphasized, only looks. But strength training, which focuses on intensity rather than repetition, helps you get into the best shape possible. It's the most effective way to improve muscle tone, lose fat, and increase your metabolic rate.

If you've ever been to a traditional track meet and observed the marathoners versus the sprinters, you've likely noticed that the marathoners have some fat and almost no muscle, while the sprinters have a lot of muscle and almost no fat. Sprinters' bodies have never been forced to adapt to the harsh and unnatural conditions that marathoners put theirs through.

Increasing intensity builds optimum health for your heart, too. This approach doesn't just make the pumping more efficient, it strengthens it. With more intensity, more blood is forced into the heart and it can hold more;

you're also building muscle. The extra blood flow causes microscopic trauma in the muscle cells inside your heart, and over the next few days as you eat and sleep, your body rebuilds the damage with additional muscle cells. You're doing exactly the same thing with your heart that you would do with a bicep: you're actually building a stronger heart that can push with more force than it used to.

Second, strength training has an impact on mental health. In the January 25, 2010, edition of *The Archives of Internal Medicine*, a study showed that women between the ages of sixty-five and seventy-five who were assigned strength training twice weekly with weights, or on exercise machines, had improved on tests of "executive function"—including planning, organizing, and strategizing—by ten to twelve percent over the course of one year. On the other hand, the mental acuity of the control group, who were assigned twice-weekly balance or toning exercise routines, declined by half a percent during the same period.

> Medical research has proven that strength training builds neurological facility both in the brain and throughout the body.

Strength training triggers production of proteins that are beneficial for brain growth.

I know a lot of men and women in their eighties who have been consistent in following strength-training protocols, and to me none of them seems to have aged at all. Even their voices are as young as they were when I met them. They live at an incredibly high level of functioning for their age.

For people with neurological problems not associated with age, occupational therapists recommend exercise programs designed to stimulate the brain. As they do more physical work, their neurological ailments tend to get correspondingly better. Even people with dyslexia can be helped that way. The fact is that your brain reacts and changes according to the stimuli you give it, and strength training offers your brain the right stimuli to thrive.

Your nervous system is the electrical system of your body. If your brain is using its neurotransmitters correctly to communicate with your muscles and other systems, you're going to be more efficient, and you're going to live longer and smarter. Consider the example of walking on one of those long people-mover strips at the airport. Suppose you walk on the strip for an hour, then jump off and try to walk normally. You would be a little uncoordinated when you got off, wouldn't you? That lack of coordination is a result of the workings of your nervous system, not your muscles.

When you're performing repetitive actions, like running on a treadmill or doing the same things over and over in an aerobics class, your brain is sending out a different message than it would be if you were exercising properly.

That message isn't to your benefit; what's happening to you is the same thing that's occurring when you get off that people mover. Your neurological and muscular systems are at odds, so instead of learning to work more smoothly together, they have been working independently, practically at cross-purposes. They're not up to new challenges because they're expecting to do the same movement over and over again and take longer to adapt to changing conditions.

Repetition can affect your mental state, too, and not just because of oxidation and the production of free radicals. Repetitive exercise can also defeat other anti-aging goals. For example, Dr. Robert B. Pompa's research suggests that walking on a treadmill for an hour lowers growth hormone and testosterone for more than a day. Short-burst, high-intensity training on the other hand elevates these hormones. Our evolutionary history proves that this approach is the way we were meant to exercise our bodies.

TWO KINDS OF ACTIONS

In kinetics, we talk about two kinds of actions, closed-chain actions and open-chain actions.

Closed-Chain Actions

Happen when the hand or foot is stationary or fixed—it's on solid ground.

A good example of a closed-chain action:

A Pull-Up

Your hands are fixed to the bar, and you have to use multiple muscles and joints to pull yourself up. Your hands, wrists, upper and lower arms, and chest are all involved.

Open-Chain Actions

Occur when the hand or foot is free to move around.

A good example of an open-chain action:

A Leg Extension

You raise and lower your leg, with or without resistance from an exercise machine. This focuses the stress against one set of muscles and joints, rather than spreading potential stress around.

Closed-chain actions are generally considered to be safer and cause fewer injuries. Walking on solid ground is a closed-chain action: your foot is in stasis (a period or state of inactivity or equilibrium) when it hits the ground. However, when you're on a treadmill (or one of those people movers), you're doing an open-chain action, because the treadmill is moving. Your foot may be in stasis relative to the treadmill, but the treadmill is still moving you along.

Our bodies are adapted to closed-chain actions because they most resemble natural human activities—such as picking something up or reaching—that require multiple muscle groups to move at the same time. When you're performing an open-chain action, only one set of muscles and joints is required, so your brain shuts everything else down. After all, if only one set of muscles is needed, why make the rest run at full speed? That's not efficient, however, because it's much better to have all muscles attuned to changes in the environment in case you're presented with an unexpected physical challenge, such as tripping on a stone.

Doing open-chain actions (such as running on a treadmill) isn't like walking up a hill, yet we use running on a treadmill as a basis for our stress tests. But you can't get a true measure of a body's stress if you're not using all the muscles. There's no harm in using a treadmill occasionally—in bad weather, for example—but it won't build your muscles the same way as running up and down hills would.

THE EFFECTS OF AGING

My brother had Parkinson's disease, which current research shows is tied closely to oxidative stress. I remember asking if he could tell me what it was like to have the disease. I wasn't trying to be cruel, and he knew that; rather he understood that I'm just a curious guy who always wants answers.

He said, "When you stand up, you think, *I'm going to take a step forward.* But for a few moments nothing happens. There's a delayed reaction because the brain and nerves aren't working together the way they should."

> **Synapse** | \\'si-ˌnaps, sə-'naps\\
> noun
> the point at which a nervous impulse passes from one neuron to another.

As most people age, it's a common problem that synapses slow down, even if a person doesn't have Parkinson's. You'll see a lot of older people walking slowly and shuffling their feet. They're afraid to take a normal step, because doing so depends on their body getting some complex instructions very quickly and then receiving immediate feedback if something unexpected happens. A split-second delay can put you on the ground in a heartbeat.

If you're not taking care of your synapses, everything will slow down as you age. This is yet another reason why physical exercise will help you stay spry, mentally alert, and able to cope efficiently with everyday activities.

MANAGING DIABETES

According to the National Institute on Health, diabetes is affecting larger and younger segments of our population, but proper strength training and professional help with your diet reduces your chances of being afflicted with the disease. When you're building muscle tissue, proteins are released that take up the glucose in your bloodstream, giving your muscles more energy and lowering your blood-glucose levels. This also helps your mental functioning.

In 2005-2008, based on fasting glucose or hemoglobin A1C levels, 35% of US adults aged 20-65 and 50% of adults aged 65 or older had pre-diabetes. Applying this percentage to the entire US population in 2010 yields an estimated 79 million American adults aged 20 years or older with pre-diabetes, which equates to 194 billion dollars in US healthcare spending.[4]

The epidemic of diabetes in the US is caused primarily by poor diets and is exacerbated by doing the wrong things to manage the disease. Patients are given oral doses of anti-diabetic medications to manage their insulin levels rather than building lean muscle mass that can naturally do so.

Understanding these fundamentals, I have had incredible success in reducing the symptoms of many former and current diabetic clients at the Duffy Fitness Institute. The healthiest people, in my opinion, run sprints and eat grass-fed, natural beef and organic fruits and vegetables. This kind of approach is good for diabetic people, too.

One thing we do right in this country is the Presidential Physical Fitness Award, which was created in 1956 by President Dwight D. Eisenhower. There are a few exercises, such as sit-ups, that should be removed from the protocol (see the next chapter), but it's quite good in general and includes sprints, pull-ups, and an agility course, which are great tests for determining health and functionality.

Exercise-wise, sprints are the best anaerobic, fast-twitch, muscle-building form of running. I believe a lot of people are more genetically inclined to be

4 "The United States of Diabetes: Challenges and Opportunities in the Decade Ahead." United Health Center for Health Reform and Modernization Working paper 5 November 2010 http://www.unitedhealthgroup.com/hrm/unh_workingpaper5.pdf

good at sprints, as they best reflect how we lived in prehistoric times. Back then, people walked between villages and saved their energy for hunting, gathering, and loving, the basic necessities of life.

When you're being trained by a professional strength and conditioning coach, everything he or she recommends focuses on improving mental and physical health through intensity.

For example, a powerlifter who hoists five hundred pounds at one time has an extremely high intensity; someone lifting a five-pound barbell does not. When you're working at an exceptionally high intensity, your brain is working at a high level too. It takes a lot of focus to lift a heavy weight—pulling every single muscle at one time in balance—and it raises your nervous system to an entirely different level. When the nervous system is running well, you significantly improve physical fitness. It's a positive feedback loop, which doesn't mean that everyone has to be a powerlifter, but rather that exercises that activate the nervous system are vital.

What we're building in our Ageless Human exercise protocols, and have used at our physical facility, are corrective exercises that stimulate both the slow- and fast-twitch muscle fibers. Some popular exercise programs do this as well; however, they tend to overstimulate the brain and may cause physical injuries. As the symptoms of aging are essentially decreases in function, we work to *increase* mental and physical function and *decrease* the symptoms of aging. This is the best anti-aging technique. Ultimately, our goal is to train our clients back to the youthful functionality they've been accustomed to when undertaking everyday activities. Through our methodologies, we promote not only longevity but a higher quality of life.

Overall, the people who are consistently healthy in mind and body are the ones who practice traditional strength training and sprints, which is what comes naturally to us as human beings. By returning to the basics of functional movement, our mental as well as physical well-being will reap the benefits.

CRITICAL TAKEAWAY

RESISTANCE STRENGTH TRAINING HAS ANTI-AGING EFFECTS THAT IMPROVE COGNITIVE AS WELL AS PHYSICAL HEALTH.

MYTH BUSTER IN MOTION

Exercise has proven benefits, not only for the body but also for the mind. Strength training improves brain function, and we recommend sequences that are challenging but not stressful on joints for upper and lower body.

- ❖ Walking lunges forward and backward
- ❖ Non-dominant hand leads in pull-downs with opposite foot balance
- ❖ Sequencing front and back opposite hand and foot with isolated functional moments

Low-intensity, repetitive exercise on machines does *not* offer the many cognitive rewards that strength training does with regard to hormonal responses, memory, and executive function.

For instructions on performing functional brain-stimulating exercises, visit our website at:

www.ageless-human.com

MYTH 3

SIT-UPS GIVE YOU SIX-PACK ABS

TRUTH:

Crunches have no effect on fat loss in the abdomen and can negatively affect your spine.

Alignment is Key:
Protecting the spine

Should You Do Sit-Ups at All?
The short answer is *no*

Balancing Your Back Exercises:
The path to better alignment

Everybody wants six-pack abs, or at least an absence of bulge around the middle. What's the best way to get those abs? Sit-ups, right? Lots of sit-ups. Wrong.

Your abs are like any other muscle; when you work them, you build them, but you don't necessarily lower your body fat. You can have abs that are rock-hard and still have a big gut covering them.

It's also possible—as with other muscles—to overdevelop them. I've seen a lot of bodybuilders who have overtrained their abdominals by doing too many reps. An excess of crunches actually creates a muscular imbalance, so bellies stick out because there's nowhere else for the muscles to go.

Many people become slaves to crunches and sit-ups when the real issue isn't their abdominal strength but their body fat. Just because you're exercising the muscles near an area with extra fat doesn't mean you'll burn that fat in particular.

Body fat is reduced through a comprehensive training program, incorporating resistance training and through clean eating and smart calorie consumption, not sit-ups.

Professionals in the fitness industry already know this. In fact, I once asked a competitive bodybuilder who had phenomenal abs what his secret was. He said he didn't do anything for his abs until about a week before the contest. Then he joked that he did four sets of nothing every day. His great abs were a result of his diet and his general training, not from doing a thousand sit-ups before breakfast.

One of my clients, a participant in the Miss California contest, had suffered a broken back years before. She needed to look her best, but she couldn't do many of the exercises I would normally recommend. I worked out an isometric exercise plan for her and had her follow a nutritional program focused on organic and natural foods (which we'll discuss in the final chapter of this book). By the time of the contest, she had beautiful abdominal muscles, but they didn't come about from exercise alone, and certainly not from sit-ups.

So if sit-ups and crunches aren't going to give you six-pack abs, what are they going to do for you? Throw your body out of alignment, that's what.

ALIGNMENT IS KEY

The number one cause of back injuries is excessive forward bending, which during exercise mainly comes from doing crunches—especially from the floor —as well as any exercise where we're pushing our bodies forward in an unnatural way.

We're seeing an epidemic of back injuries in America—even in people who don't do a lot of crunches—that often stem from leaning forward all day over our keyboards and smartphones. Sixty to sixty-five percent of the general public suffers disc herniations to some degree, even if most don't know it yet. Before you develop a noticeable problem, you've probably spent years abusing your back.

At some point this curvature will worsen to the point where you can't straighten up fully. That's when major back injuries occur. All of a sudden, out of nowhere, you'll do something in a far-forward bending position —perhaps picking up your child or simply leaning over the sink to brush your teeth—and you'll experience excruciating pain that will send you to the doctor. He or she will give you drugs to help reduce the pain, and if they don't work, they'll send you to physical therapy. If that doesn't work, you'll undergo surgery and think: *Man, brushing my teeth is no good for me.*

> Think about it: If you're constantly bending forward, you're working against gravity and straining your back.

I'm kidding, of course. But the damage is really a result of those years and years of abuse from leaning forward. And if you're doing a lot of sit-ups and crunches on the floor, you'll be doing that much more abuse to your spine, and faster.

Trust me, I've suffered for exactly those reasons.

SIT-UPS FLATTEN YOUR BACK

Hurting your lower back is only one of the disadvantages of doing sit-ups and crunches; it also shortens the front part of your body, or the *anterior*. If you continually do too many crunches, particularly on the floor, what will happen to you is what happened to me—my anterior muscles threw my back out of alignment because I frequently leaned much further forward than I normally would.

I don't care how good your form is, if you're doing crunches on the floor, you're going to shorten the muscles that connect your hips to your abdominals—your hip flexors—and it will flatten out your lower back.

To see what shape your spine is in, stand with your back against the wall and your heels touching the wall. If you don't have a space between your back and the wall, your back is flat. But the back should have a nice, big S-curve to it. The spine works, or should work, as a spring, which helps your spinal cord resist the compression of vertebrae that occurs when you walk or run. It should be able to move up and down easily. Of course, this important human spring may be compressed in an unhealthy way, and that affects height and flexibility. But with sit-ups and crunches, it's the opposite problem: your spring is being stretched straight.

When your back is flat, your vertebrae prevent your spinal cord from moving freely without being pinched. It's easy, without realizing it, to damage your spine and spinal cord to the point where, after a number of years, you lean forward and hurt yourself by doing something as simple as making the bed or stepping off the curb. Back injuries are insidious. They creep in, occurring over a long period of time.

Here's what we've seen as a typical client's exercise protocol:

- ❖ Push-ups
- ❖ Sit-ups
- ❖ Run six or seven miles

Honestly, they could not pick a worse protocol to get healthy.

Those exercises pull their weight forward over their center of gravity and flatten the curve of their lower backs.

I used to be the king of sit-ups. I've probably done a half-million in my life. I ran a lot, too, and I tried to run with a perfectly flat back. All the force that would normally be distributed throughout my body was being focused in my lower back. That's how I ended up in a wheelchair. So much for my pride in my flat back.

SIT-UPS STRAIN YOUR NECK

Possibly even worse than the strain on your back is the strain that sit-ups place on your neck.

When doing a sit-up, most of us put our hands behind our heads, using our arms to help pull ourselves up. That means we're putting force on the back of the neck every time we do a sit-up, jerking our head forward, over and over again. Not only are you giving yourself a minor case of whiplash doing this, but over time you'll pull the bones in your neck out of alignment. Your head will go too far forward on a permanent basis, and the muscles on the front of your neck will shorten, which starts a vicious cycle: your head goes further forward, your muscles shorten more, and so on.

Again, you're taking the curve out of your spine. Your head is meant to be balanced on your shoulders, which means there should be a slight backward curve to your neck. When you hold your head forward, that curve unbends itself, taking the spring out and adding compression.

When you do a lot of sit-ups and crunches, your body will begin to look like the Leaning Tower of Pisa. We're not built to walk around like that, so it's only a matter of time before your back or neck is affected negatively.

SHOULD YOU DO SIT-UPS AT ALL?

I would have to say no, because most of us have forward-leaning postures already, and sit-ups only exacerbate that tendency. I haven't done sit-ups for five years and yet I still have well-developed abs. There are many other beneficial exercises you could be doing other than sit-ups or crunches, ones that don't damage you structurally and that keep your body balanced. You can visit our website for some examples.

The secret of developing your abs is to focus beyond your rectus abdominis muscles, the ones that help you do sit-ups and keep your gut from pushing out of your abdomen when you lift weights. There are layers and layers of muscles underneath the rectus abdominis muscles, and we're not working them enough.

The key muscles in abdominal development are the transverse abdominis muscles—the really deep muscles that are integral to your abdominal wall. They act as a muscular girdle around the abdomen, helping us keep our balance. And, as we've learned, becoming unbalanced by constantly leaning forward doesn't do anybody any good. The transverse abdominis muscles are crucial to many of our basic functions, including breathing, bending, pulling, pushing, twisting, having sex, running at top speed, and more.

These core muscles are so deep that sit-ups and crunches aren't going to build them. You have to develop them by causing some kind of instability in your center of gravity using tension or weight, or by adding speed. Some exercises that are good for the transverse abdominis muscles include squats, dead lifts, and lunges, all of which lend to developing core strength.

BALANCING YOUR BACK

If you're leaning forward, you need to spend more time lengthening the front of your body and shortening the back, which will strengthen your back and glute muscles and help improve your posture in general. You don't want to go too far and become unbalanced the other way, but considering how much we tend to lean forward, that's hard to do.

To build strength in your back, you need to do more pulling exercises. When you pull something toward you, you have to pull your shoulders back, and your whole back has to support that movement. Pulling is an activity that comes naturally to us as humans. Sit-ups aren't.

To make a change in your muscles (using intensity), you're going to have to use weight.

Some examples of pulling exercises are:

❖ Pull-downs

❖ Pull-ups

❖ Low pulley rows

❖ One-armed rows

❖ Bent-over rows (a.k.a. barbell rows)

Anything you pull is going to strengthen your back. Because we're already doing too much leaning forward, you want to minimize the pushing exercises that you do. Anyone who uses the bench press for the majority of his or her workout is going to have problems.

Here are some other possibilities:

① One of the ways to minimize pushing is to lie on a ball while you're pushing, so you're actually using your lower back to help make the movement work.

② Another way to work in some length to your abdominals is to lie on top of a Swiss ball (the kind of large exercise ball you can use to sit at your desk) on your back, put your arms over your head, and stay in that position for a while. For the most part, people find that it feels really good, because they're finally getting some stretch to their abdominals.

③ Yoga does a pretty good job of stretching your abdominals with cobras (lying on the floor on your stomach and lifting your upper body off the floor), bows (lying on the floor on your stomach and holding your ankles), and downward dogs (getting on your hands and feet with your glutes as far up in the air as they'll go).

④ At the Duffy Fitness Institute, we've developed another method of strengthening your core with a Swiss ball: simply put your hands on top of the ball and roll forward onto it. This lengthens the stomach and strengthens it at the same time. The posture actually isolates the stomach. It's an effective way of strengthening your abs that doesn't involve doing crunches and sit-ups. You're in a safe position because you're higher off the ground, so your back won't be subjected to overstraining.

If your abdominals aren't strong, and you don't train them correctly, it will impact you throughout your life. Whether they're too weak or too strong, you're going to have problems.

Your motor reflexes change to help protect you from the daily consequences of being constantly out of alignment, taking stress from your back. In the short term this can have a positive effect, but it will have a negative domino effect on other muscles over time.

When you hurt your back, a lot of times the glutes will shut down to prevent you from doing further damage to yourself. If you push yourself past the pain, you may hurt yourself badly. For example, a lot of professional athletes who get injured will take painkillers so they can get back on the field. Because they're pushing past the natural feedback (pain) their bodies are giving them, they turn minor injuries into major ones.

You're supposed to listen to pain. When you're in pain, stop what you're doing to prevent more injury. If you mask the pain, you might be able to go out and perform for a while longer, but you're guaranteed to subject yourself to further injury.

Remember, we're still built the same way, more or less, as our long-ago ancestors, even though we live in a far different world. Your survival instincts are essentially the same and your body's response to injury is as well. If exercises aren't right for you, it is irrelevant whether you're doing them correctly or not.

I recently met with a high-level golf coach who told me that the first part of education is not to tell people what to do and how to do it, but to tell people why they should perform certain actions. If you only know *how*, you may forget the action, change your mind, or procrastinate. When you know the *why*, you won't change your mind and quit.

That's why this book is focusing on teaching you the *why* underlying our recommendations, rather than providing detailed exercise protocols; those you can find on our website and videos. Yet most exercise routines are focused on the mechanics rather than the reasons for the routine. Exercising properly isn't something you can do on autopilot. You have to understand the logic behind the activity or you're going to wind up injuring yourself.

You've been hearing all your life how to do sit-ups and crunches correctly, but you haven't heard a word of why you should or shouldn't be doing them in the first place. We're working hard, but we're not working smart. You have to approach exercise with your brain, from a whole-body perspective.

The American public is starting to get smarter and beginning to question whether or not, for example, a person with great abs actually got them by using a piece of expensive, trendy equipment. Maybe the person demonstrating the equipment developed those abs using some other method years ago and recently went on an extreme diet to make them stand out. Some people may have been born with the potential for great abs. They may be former athletes. They may be using chemicals and drugs to make themselves look leaner. They may just employ a good airbrush artist. We don't know.

It's healthy to be skeptical about appearances so that we learn to do the exercises that work best for our own bodies and minds.

Yet there are still people with forty-eight-inch waistlines who think they can lie on their backs on the floor, jerk their heads forward to their knees a few thousand times, get up and run with a hundred extra pounds on their bodies, and transform themselves. They can't. They are only hurting themselves.

If you've been steered toward the wrong exercises your whole life, it's not your fault. My recommendation is always to minimize machine training and concentrate on an individualized program—one that focuses on supporting and strengthening body structure, alignment, and stability.

In seeking out the best possible fitness plan, be sure to find one that is right for you as an individual. Assess its advantages and drawbacks for your particular body. I believe that if you understand the *why* of exercise, you'll be able to make proper decisions and get healthy.

CRITICAL TAKEAWAY

ELIMINATE SIT-UPS AND MINIMIZE MACHINE TRAINING, CONCENTRATING INSTEAD ON FUNCTIONAL MOVEMENT PATTERNS.

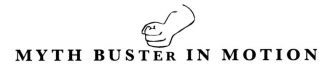

MYTH BUSTER IN MOTION

Though it goes against years of improper guidance we've all received, core-building exercises that target visceral fat should be your only focus for stronger abs.

Try:

- Dead lifts
- Squats
- Sprints
- Supine lateral ball rolls
- Single-leg jackknife sit-ups
- Swiss ball crunches
- Pullovers
- Straight-arm lat pulldowns

For instructions on how to perform these and other core-building exercises, visit our website at:

www.ageless-human.com

MYTH 4

THE ONLY PURPOSE OF EXERCISE IS TO LOOK BETTER

TRUTH:

Training for looks won't increase stamina, flexibility, strength, or function.

- **How Aerobic Exercise Makes You Look Worse:**
  The silent damage

- **How Exercise Machines Work:**
  The hidden truth

- **Functional Movement Patterns:**
  Look *and* feel better

Wanting to look good is a decent enough motivation to get on the path to health; anything that rouses you from apathy has to get some credit. But "looking good" isn't a healthy goal to set for yourself for training.

Think about people who love to tan. They start out wanting to look good, but over time their skin turns leathery and wrinkled. Because they put the goal of "looking good" first, they've actually lessened their attractiveness and increased their risk of skin cancer.

You can make the same argument about exercise: by focusing on appearance, you may end up looking worse than you did when you started, not to mention risking your health.

The focus on good looks reached a zenith during the bodybuilding craze of the sixties and seventies. Men bought every bodybuilding magazine available and followed everything those self-described experts in the magazines told them to do, leaving most of them injured. At best they found themselves on up-and-down cycles of loss and gain, rather than achieving consistent results. Same with the aerobics craze, as we've discussed.

Think about what makes people attractive:

❖ They look healthy.
❖ They look young.
❖ They look firm and fit.

A strong resemblance to a starvation victim with bad posture doesn't make you attractive. Stiff, exhausted, muscle-bound people don't look good either. Trust me when I tell you to forget about looks.

If you focus on functionality, your body will be healthier—which means it will look healthier and you'll feel younger.

Charles Poliquin says:

At any given gym or fitness center, the one thing I notice is that people who do the same workout month after month, year after year, often continue to look the same as before, or worse. These people think they're doing what they need to do to achieve their goals, but they aren't. When I ask them what they want to get out of that workout, they usually tell me that they're trying to lose weight. I ask them how long they've been doing the workout, and most say they've followed that same routine somewhere between six and twelve months, with thirty to sixty minutes of training per workout, five times a week. But they look the same or worse than when they began.

THE RIGHT EXERCISES FOR YOUR BODY TYPE

I once trained a family of swimmers. One of the sons had a long, lean body and was an excellent swimmer; however, some preliminary tests convinced me he was an even better sprinter. His ability on the track was incredible. I told his family that if he trained correctly, he could get into the Olympics. His strength was undeniable.

I put him on a weight-training program, which was considered taboo at the time. The theory was that too much muscle mass would make the swimmer less streamlined and therefore slower; nobody was doing it. One of the most widely known swim coaches at the time made a threatening phone call telling me "not to bulk up that kid." But we kept going, and after three to six months, his speed increased amazingly. He tried out for the Olympics and made it as an alternate.

This is what I mean about choosing the exercises that suit your body type and that increase functionality, rather than following random programs that may be right for someone else, but not for you.

HOW EXERCISE MACHINES MAKE YOU LOOK GOOD BUT DIMINISH YOUR FUNCTION

When you walk into a typical gym, you see a very small area dedicated to free weights and an enormous area filled with cardio and other types of equipment. Naturally, you as a beginner assume that you need to spend more time on each of the machines than anything else.

So you get on the weight machines and pull things up and down, then move to the cardio equipment and run for twenty minutes or so on a treadmill. You believe you *must* be getting into shape. If you weight train on a machine, you're likely to do leg extensions. So you sit down, hook your feet into a contraption, and pull them straight up and down. As a result, you *will* develop the muscles in your thighs; there's no question about it. Over a period of time, even if you don't know what you're doing, you're going to get visible results.

But what happens after you get off the machine? You leave the gym and take the escalator down to the parking lot. If you're driving, you open the car door, take a long stride in with your right leg, balance your weight, then pull your left leg in and sit down. The movement is a side lateral lunge combined with a squat. Your thighs are strong, but getting into your car doesn't demand that you move your legs straight up and down; only the muscles associated with squats and lunges do that.

The leg extension you're doing on the machine, even though it develops your thigh, isn't going to transfer over to a lunge-and-squat combination very well. One, you're not working any hamstrings when you do the leg extensions; and two, the movement pattern is completely different. This is especially true if you drive an SUV or some kind of truck where you have to step up.

Bottom line, that up-and-down strength is not going to benefit you when it comes to everyday tasks.

Good trainers and strength coaches will train you relative to the kinds of actions you do naturally in life.

For example, when your trainer has you do squats, it's not for the purpose of developing your ability to put weight on your back and lift it up and down. He or she is training you to reflect movements like going to the bathroom or getting into your car.

One of the shortcomings of using the machines is that you're not using the full spectrum of the muscles of your entire body the way they're meant to work. Using those machines occasionally, once you get your body in shape, is a different story; you can develop great-looking thighs using them. But those people may hurt themselves doing activities that require whole-body strength.

Another problem is that machine work may unbalance you structurally. Let's say you're doing a lot of leg extensions but not much hamstring work. You're going to end up with knee problems. Nearly every time a person comes into the gym with knee issues, the underlying problem is weak hamstrings.

Obviously, if you do all that work on your thighs without following up with a good hamstring exercise, that machine isn't really helping you at all. It's setting you up for injury.

Most people don't like to do squats or lunges, which is understandable. One, it takes significant effort to do them effectively; two, there are not enough good trainers or exercise physiologists around to teach people the correct way of doing them; and three, it's tempting to do other exercises instead of squats and lunges because people would rather do exercises that don't wear them out so quickly.

But I believe that if you can read a book or listen to an audiobook and exercise at the same time, you're not exercising effectively. If you don't focus on what you're doing physically, you're not taxing yourself enough and you're risking injury from lack of attention.

Let's turn our focus again to functionality.

ACHIEVING OPTIMUM FUNCTIONALITY

I took a trip to China and found that, in general, Chinese people are pretty functional. They can do things that Americans can't do at all, like sit on their heels, because they practice those things on a consistent basis and because they use squat toilets, which are basically a hole in the floor with a flush mechanism. To get off the floor from a squat toilet takes a tremendous amount of abdominal strength.

In the United States, toilets are being designed to be taller and taller, and there are more handrails in bathrooms. Why? Because we can't do squats and are becoming less agile. This isn't a comfortable subject to talk about, but Americans are losing their basic functionality in this regard. It's such an epidemic among older adults that we're coming to think of it as normal.

If you can't sit on your heels or use a squat toilet, you've got a problem, because your abdominals aren't working the way they should. I truly believe there's a correlation between the lack of functional training (especially with squats) and the American epidemic of incontinence.

If your abdominal muscles aren't working, you're going to lose a lot of ability to control your bowel movements, too. That's why many people get injured in the bathroom from straining too hard, because the extent of their abdominal work (if they do any at all) is a sit-up, which is useless when it comes to squatting. Sit-ups won't strengthen all the muscles you need to control your abdomen, rather they only serve to help you curl forward, which is not what you want to do in a squat at all.

Some certification programs will tell you that it's really bad to go past the point where your thighs are parallel with the floor, yet anyone who has used a Western toilet can tell you that most of them cause you to do exactly that.

You sit in that position, and then you must get up again. It's getting to the point where people who are supposedly without disabilities have to use a handrail in order to sit down and stand up again on a Western toilet.

I estimate that about twenty-five percent of our clients with back pain have also had problems going to the toilet. Many have also triggered back pain as they stood up, blowing their backs out, because they had no strength in that position.

EXERCISING FOR FUNCTIONALITY

If you rely strictly on machine training, you're working the primary movers—the muscles that provide the main part of the work—but you're not working out the stabilizers and the neutralizers.

Stabilizers | stā-bə-ˌlī-zərs
noun (pl)
the muscles that keep one part of your body immobile while another part is moving.

Stabilizers align your bones to prevent damage.

Neutralizers | ˈnü-trə-ˌlī-zərs
noun (pl)
elements that prevent unwanted muscle motions.

**Neutralizers, for example, keep the foot from
rolling outward while running.**

If you're constantly sitting on a workout machine, all you're going to work is the prime-mover muscles. There is no need for stabilization when you're on a machine, because the machine provides the stabilization for you.

For example, if you sit on a bench to do leg extensions, then get off the bench and try to squat up and down, you'll realize that squats use more muscles and in a more concerted way, too, than the exercise you've just been doing. With squats, you have to use your stabilizers and neutralizers to help support your big muscles and make sure you don't tip over.

Bodybuilders and other athletes experience many muscle tears because they spend a lot of time working their primary muscles and don't work their stabilizing and neutralizing muscles enough. Another reason is that some of them use steroids, a side effect of which is that it's easy to tear a muscle. People get so excited about putting muscle on in a hurry that they overdevelop the prime-mover muscles to the point where the stabilizers and neutralizers can't hold the joint steady. The joint moves the wrong way and muscle rips.

> You can look good by doing isolated exercises on machines, but if that's primarily what you do for exercise, you're going to have a problem. At some point you'll hurt yourself.

By training for functionality first, you will naturally look better than you would if you trained for appearance first. You'll be lean and able to function better, with fewer injuries, for the rest of your life. And you *will* burn calories!

A recent study in *Medicine & Science in Sports & Exercise*[5] shows that the calories you burn after an exercise session are increased for at least a day and possibly up to two days, but only if you do high-intensity workouts. In the study, people who exercised for about forty-five minutes at seventy percent of their max VO$_2$—or maximum capability to use oxygen during exercise—burned about 460 calories during the exercise (bike riding), and an additional 190 calories throughout the day, as opposed to studies on the same people on a non-exercise day. People who exercised for forty-five minutes at only fifty percent of their VO$_2$ max, however, didn't have any additional calorie burn.

The VO$_2$ max of the sprinter and the average person who does sprint work (or intensity workouts with weights) is increased every single time by between fourteen and twenty-eight percent.

---

[5] Knab et al. "A 45-minute Vigorous Exercise Bout Increases Metabolic Rate for 19 hours," *Medicine & Science in Sports & Exercise* 43 (May 2011): 266.

For individuals who want to lose a large amount of weight, I've found the best method is interval training. This involves bursts of high-intensity work interspersed with intervals of low-intensity work. I suggest to clients that they forget about running except for sprints—although those who are heavy should avoid sprint work until they lose some weight.

I recommend that people cycle through two or more quick exercises back to back, going through the series of exercises as one rep then moving to the next rep with as little rest as possible. It's what we call circuit training, and it's so intense that it causes your body to burn calories for up to forty-eight hours after your workout. It increases the strength of your lungs and heart, too.

We've been doing the same functional movement patterns over and over since primitive times. In fact, Paul Chek of the CHEK Institute trademarked a system of primal patterns. The movements include:

❖ Squats
❖ Lunges
❖ Bends
❖ Pushes

❖ Pulls
❖ Twists
❖ Gaits (walking, jogging, running)

Because they're the actions we do every day, it's important for anybody who wants to maintain their functionality to practice every single one of these on a consistent basis. These are the same actions that our ancestors had to perform in order to survive.

Functional training comes into play every day. When you get out of bed, you lean forward and put your feet on the ground: it's a like a one-legged squat. When you get in the shower, you bend forward and backward to wash yourself. You squat when you sit at your desk and when you get up again. You pull the refrigerator open; you push it shut. You pull things out of your car trunk; you push them into place. You twist when you turn around to get something out of the back seat of the car. You pick things up off the floor. You lift things over your head to put them away. You use your gait all day, moving from place to place.

The aforementioned exercises are clearly not obscure ones that have no practical applications in real life, yet our fitness routine still tends to support that we'll need to do a leg extension, for example, like we do on a machine.

But how often does that come up? Once a year, when your doctor checks your reflexes? On the contrary, functional exercises help us achieve our maximum potential in everyday life activities.

SEX

Another functional movement that's near to our hearts is sex. We've already discussed the way aerobic exercise can dampen production of hormones and depress your libido, so let's stick with strength training, shall we?

An active sex life will work your abdominal muscles hard. Sometimes after sex, you'll wake up the next day and say, "My lower abs are sore," and that reflects the work you've put into your transverse abdominis muscles.

With sex, you have a lot of intensity and speed going on, so it's vital to be able to stabilize your abdomen, and that means coordinating your transverse abdominis muscles and your core muscles.

Obviously, you must have an active, fit core in order to have great sex.

If your abdominal muscles aren't strong and your back is weak, you're not going to be a good lover or last very long. I don't care how much Viagra you take, you won't to be able to keep up the pace, or anything else, in the bedroom.

This lack of core strength is a primary reason why there are a lot of injuries in the bedroom. There's no difference between trying to lift a heavy weight before you're ready for it than trying to pull a marathon in the bedroom when you're not fit—and that goes equally for men and women. You can do even more damage to yourself in the bedroom than during a workout at the gym; the emotion and endorphins produced during sex will help mask any injuries. You'll keep going and not know what you've done to yourself until later.

Injuring yourself in the bedroom is pretty common. People don't want to talk about it because it's an embarrassing subject. But the better shape you're in functionally, with lower body fat and a brain that's working on a high level, the better sex you're going to have.

> Making love starts with your brain, and if you've numbed it by doing repetitive sit-ups and stressing it with aerobic exercise, you and your partner will pay the price.

When I had my back injury, I asked my doctor what I should do about sex. He said, "Make love on your back." But that didn't help. When I consulted a fitness expert, he said, "If you have sex on your back, you're lifting a hundred and twenty pounds up and down. If you don't have a proper curve to your spine, it's only going to hurt you."

Historically, we recognized very early on that having good abdominal strength is vital to good sex. For thousands of years, people in the Indian tradition have been using tantric techniques during sex to control their abdominals and lower back, and to improve function in the prostate area through breathing.

BREATHING

Your abs also control your respiratory functions. If your abs aren't working at a high level, you're not going to be able to breathe correctly. People with weak abs and backs breathe through their chests, because they don't have the strength to draw the air all the way down, as a singer or martial artist might. Sprinters, powerlifters, and yoga masters know how to use their breath to add functionality and reduce the stress that they put on their bodies.

To summarize, our bodies weren't designed to operate aerobically for long periods of time on a daily basis, nor were they designed for certain muscles to operate in isolation.

We live in three dimensions; we don't usually just move in the straight forward-straight back motions that fitness machines impose on us.

Instead, you're constantly moving in primal patterns, either singly or combined. If you can't do these things without pain, you're not going to be able to make it through life very well.

The majority of accidents happen outside your strength area. For most people this means bending to the side or twisting. They'll tell you that they hurt their back reaching around for something in the back seat or turning to grab an object that wasn't even heavy. I know how those people exercise: when they're at the gym they move from machine to machine, then they hit the treadmill for twenty minutes.

A prime example lies in a bodybuilder who came to me with huge arms and legs. Not long afterward I heard that he'd ripped his bicep. How? Bending over to open his garage door. He was trying to pull the door up and it stuck, so he yanked it, using part of his biceps that he had never used on a consistent basis. He was so used to flexing his fist up to his shoulder, over and over again, that he couldn't lift his garage door without hurting himself.

I know it's going to take some thought and work to change your routine. Unlike sitting on a machine and moving a bar in and out, functional training involves intelligence and balance, not just strength. However, you will end up far more functional, better looking, and better in bed, than you would by following what has come to be standard and highly ineffective workout routines.

CRITICAL TAKEAWAY

AVOID TRENDY QUICK FIXES IN FAVOR OF UNDERSTANDING THE SCIENCE BEHIND YOUR EXERCISE.

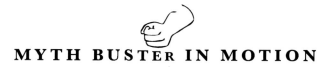

MYTH BUSTER IN MOTION

Looking better is great, but that gift can only come through fitness that truly makes you *feel* better first. The combination of functional exercises and proper nutrition is the key to enhance longevity and increase the quality of life. As such, we recommend functional exercises that focus on replicating the movement in everyday life:

❖ Squatting   ❖ Pushing

❖ Lunging   ❖ Pulling

❖ Bending   ❖ Twisting

For exercises that use basic movement patterns or for further instruction on those listed, visit our website at:

www.ageless-human.com

Note: Use of proper supplements is also paramount to a healthy inner and outer appearance. These recommendations are detailed in the Notes on Nutrition section in the back of the book.

MYTH 5

WOMEN SHOULDN'T WEIGHT TRAIN

> **TRUTH:**
> Women need MORE strength training for toning,
> fat loss, and function.

Ⓧ Why Women Should Train for More Muscle:
Immunity, longevity, and burning of fat

Ⓧ How to Train for Muscle:
Interval training

A common myth is that women shouldn't weight train, because if they were to so much as pick up a pair of dumbbells or barbells, they would "bulk up" and lose their feminine shape. A typical belief is that women should stick with cardio, toning, Pilates, or balance work, when in fact women who weight train don't lose their feminine appearance at all. Except in rare cases, genetically speaking, they can't develop huge, bulging muscles because they don't have enough testosterone in their genetic composition to look like a man.

Testosterone synthesizes proteins to rebuild muscle fibers. Women do have some testosterone produced by their ovaries, but an average woman has eight to ten times less testosterone than a man. Logically, it's going to be eight to ten times as much work for her to produce the equivalent amount of muscle mass. So if a guy lifts two hundred pounds, a woman would have to lift two thousand pounds to get the same amount of muscle. That's not going to happen.

Bodybuilding women get big because they take a lot of testosterone or testosterone-related products called steroids. Of course, a few women do build muscle easily due to high natural levels of testosterone, but they tend to find this out early on and put it to good use, such as playing professional sports. In forty years of training, I've seen only five women (other than professional athletes) with that kind of genetic predisposition.

Muscles are so dependent on testosterone that when men get older and their testosterone levels drop, they lose muscle, particularly if they don't do any strength training. After your fifties, it can take extra effort to keep muscle on your body. For women of any age, it's even harder, and it takes a serious professional strategy. A woman will never have to worry about accidentally bulking up too much.

So if building strength isn't going to bulk women up, what are the benefits of weight training?

ACID BUFFERING

The more muscle and bone mass you have, the greater acid buffering power you possess. The theory is that—similar to oxidation reactions—acids, which have a positive electrical charge, bind to other molecules easily, disrupting systems throughout your body.

Research suggests that acidity can be buffered with protein, potassium, magnesium, and calcium, so having extra amounts of these elements in your bones and muscles help keep your body less acidic and more balanced. Your immune system will also be much stronger, and you'll have a better chance of surviving diseases, from swine flu to cancer.

I've seen a lot of women, especially in Hollywood, become vegans and lose all their muscle, which can be catastrophic. If you lose a lot of muscle and can't get your body to a balanced state, your metabolic system is going to start stripping the acid neutralizers it needs in the form of calcium from your bones.

An acidic imbalance is also going to lower your endurance. Women who do a lot of long-distance running or take frequent, long aerobics classes are likely to get sick more often because their immune system can't keep up. Furthermore, they're more susceptible to injuries, because they're straining their joints while weakening their bones at the same time. This issue becomes more problematic after menopause as there is higher risk of bone weakness.

LONGEVITY

A great study done recently at Tufts University (www.tufts.edu/articles/power-play) showed that the more muscle a woman puts on her body, the longer she is likely to live.

**In fact, the number one marker for longevity
in a woman is muscle.**

It is even more important than her cholesterol level or blood pressure. And the number two marker for longevity is strength—which comes from muscle.

As women get older, the more muscle they have, the easier it is for them to control their insulin and prevent metabolic syndrome, a group of risk factors that occur together and increase the risk for heart disease, stroke, and adult-onset diabetes. These factors include high blood pressure, high-fasting blood sugar, a large waist, low levels of good (HDL) cholesterol, and high levels of triglycerides in the blood from eating too much starchy or fatty food.

BURNING FAT

The more muscle you have, the easier it is to reduce body fat. Muscle burns calories faster, and strength training builds muscle.

A few of the fashion models I used to train challenged my methods at first. "Don't get me bulked up," they'd say. My response was always, "Here's the deal. You can have more muscle, or you can keep the fat." The fact is, for every extra pound of muscle you gain, you burn an extra fifty calories a day.

When I was studying in Europe, we completed a study showing that for every kilo of lean (muscle) tissue a woman gains, there was an equal loss of body fat. Let's say a woman weighs one hundred and thirty-two pounds with twenty percent body fat—or 26.5 pounds of fat. If she gains nine pounds of muscle mass, then she also loses nine pounds of fat. Now her body-fat percentage will be about thirteen percent, and the bonus is she'll look better.

A woman who worked for us at the Center went from twenty-three percent body fat to thirteen percent in about seventy days. In her case, she didn't lose a pound—she lost inches.

The more muscle a woman adds, the leaner she will look. In addition, she'll likely live a lot longer and be much more functional. Instead of focusing on bikes and treadmills, it's imperative to get stronger every year you're around.

HOW TO TRAIN FOR MUSCLE

The best way to train to build muscle, in men *and* women, is circuit training. Of course, with women, it's even more important to train correctly and maximize their workouts, because it takes a lot more work to build and maintain muscle. You don't want to be training six hours a day! With circuit training you can obtain results doing shorter, more intense workouts, thus *minimizing your time and maximizing your results.*

> **Circuit Training** | ˈsər-kət ˈtrā-niŋ
> noun
> consists of a series of short, fast exercises, one after the other, with multiple reps and multiple sets of reps.

For example, let's say you're going to do a lower-body workout with a squat, a lunge, and then a dead lift. You would take all three exercises and cycle through them, doing fifteen reps of all three for your first set, ten reps per leg on the second, and end at twenty-five reps. Basically, after each set, you would allow a short resting interval followed by a larger number of repetitions.

The speed of the movement is important. One thing that Charles Poliquin and Ian King—both world-renowned strength coaches—taught me was that you have to lower and raise the weight at certain speeds.

In our example, most of the reps are going to be two or three seconds of lowering the weight with no rest, then raising the weight quickly. Do your fifteen reps, wait ten seconds, and go on to the next set. You can do two or three exercises during a ten-second rep. At that speed, you'll definitely be breathing hard, and you'll feel a burn.

The burn comes from lactic acid, which is one of the body's good oxidation reactions; it allows your body to generate more energy quickly from fat, among other things. If you "feel the burn," you're literally feeling calories melt, and staying in the fat-burning zone is critical for your success. You probably won't get that with most types of exercise, because they're not as intense as strength training. Bear in mind that I'm talking about *burn*, not *pain*.

When most women come into a fitness center, I find that they haven't been putting their exercises together in a way that gets them to the fat-burning zone.

Most women want to work their glutes and legs; the lower-body routine I just gave as an example is the perfect way to do that.

By doing three sets of reps—with each set increasing over the last, then resting about two or three minutes, and doing three sets of reps again—and committing to three or four of those cycles twice a week, say Tuesdays and Fridays, you'll have a heck of a workout with great results over time.

It takes a while to get used to these workouts. You might feel a little nauseated at

> As women age, it's absolutely critical that they engage in a weight-training program.

first, but you can add weights as your conditioning improves. After each workout, you'll burn fat for the next day or two, as we discussed, and you'll feel much healthier.

Women come into our center with flabby arms because they've lost muscle; they likewise approach the center because they're losing functionality in their bodies, falling more often and breaking brittle bones, and losing their mental sharpness. And yet they avoid weight training for fear that they're going to look less ladylike—or at least, less like the skinny, bony kind of child-woman model that's popular these days.

Believe me, men like women with good muscle tone. Women who desire to look and feel younger and are physically able to lift weights should strength train. In fact, they have to if they want to keep their functionality and youthful appearance. Strength training is a much more effective way to build functionality than running on a treadmill or doing aerobics.

Weight training is an anti-aging protocol for women that will help balance hormones, keep the body toned and in functional shape, improve cognition, and add years to their lives.

CRITICAL TAKEAWAY

A GOOD WEIGHT-TRAINING PROGRAM FOR WOMEN MUST INCORPORATE APPROPRIATE WEIGHT VOLUME, REST, INTENSITY, REPETITIONS, TEMPO, AND SETS.

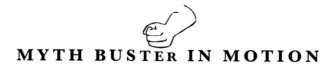

MYTH BUSTER IN MOTION

Strength training has huge anti-aging effects for women. Resistance weight training—in combination with high-intensity workouts—produces fat loss, balances cortisol and insulin, and elevates HGH and testosterone, which helps skin elastin and energy, and promotes better cognitive function.

We recommend high-intensity training where you're elevating your heart rate and exceeding expectations in lifting weight:

❖ Include weights you can lift fairly comfortably only 8-12 times.

❖ Do *not* include weights you can lift 20 times or more.

❖ Use a combination of multi-joint exercises, such as dead lifts, squats, or even sprints.

Note: This kind of training needs to be supervised by experts and a complete evaluation should be conducted before initiating this program. See the back of the book for information on professional evaluations.

MYTH 6

WEIGHT-LOSS FOCUS IS A WINNING STRATEGY

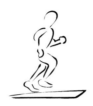

TRUTH:

Focus on fat loss while retaining and building lean muscle.

Losing Body Fat Instead of Weight:
Reduce damage to system

Types of Fat:
Understanding leads to reduction

Losing Fat for the Over-Fifty Crowd:
Not as tough as you may think

What Exercises Should You Be Doing?
Strength training, of course

In this country we seem to believe that people who are heavy should simply run a lot and stop eating as much to get healthy. We judge people's health by how much they weigh, and weight loss is celebrated regardless of the underlying health of the individual. The greatest example of that kind of mentality is the TV show *The Biggest Loser*.

For many people, egged on by programs like these, weight loss becomes a race. They ask, "How fast can I lose five hundred pounds?" instead of, "How can I permanently lose body fat in the healthiest way?"

I don't like the name of the show. *The Biggest Loser.* I find it negative and condescending toward the contestants. On the show, they talk a little bit about fat loss, but the focus is on losing weight, no matter where it comes from. That's why the contestants do an incredible amount of work on treadmills and elliptical machines.

Yes, if you do those things, you'll lose weight—especially for the first six to eight weeks or so. That also happens when you starve yourself. However, you will also lose a good deal of the muscle you've built up over the years.

Most of these contestants don't have the muscle to lose in the first place. What's more, these "losers" often deal with a lot of dangerous aftereffects. If your body loses too much water too quickly, for example, you could die.

The Biggest Loser is just one of many TV shows that focuses on losing weight, along with the drumbeat of commercials for weight-loss products. I can practically hear people out there saying, "Yeah, eventually I want to build muscle, but first I have to lose the weight." They get into this extreme weight-loss mode, planning to build up muscle later. But that's not what happens.

By destroying muscle, you're moving yourself backward—not forward. You must work to build muscle *before* you burn the fat. Focusing on losing the weight first will set you back a long, long time. Doing so is unhealthy and puts a strain on your body and its systems.

> By losing a massive amount of weight all at once, you get on a roller-coaster ride of weight swings and poor health because your metabolic rate is forever compromised.

Losing "weight" as a priority suggests that what happens to your bones, muscle, and organs—including skin—is irrelevant. Not so. For a while you may look good, but you're sure to become less functional if you lose muscle. If you train to be functional, however, you're naturally going to look good.

Of course, what people really want to lose is body fat. I believe if we focused on preserving precious muscle and other tissues as much as losing body fat, we'd have a lot fewer health problems in this country.

LOSING BODY FAT INSTEAD OF WEIGHT

Many doctors, especially when it comes to their female patients, have a problem comprehending the difference between losing body fat and simply shedding pounds. You step on a scale, you get marked off on a chart, and the doctor tells you that you need to lose X number of pounds.

If they think about body-fat percentages at all, they'll tell women that a normal level is eighteen to twenty-two percent (where a guy "should" be at fourteen to sixteen percent—though I personally believe that twelve percent body fat is a healthy percentage). However, that number is based on thin women who don't do weight training. A woman who does weight training can safely get a lot lower than that. She'll appear very lean and be extremely healthy at fourteen or fifteen percent body fat.

Our norms are completely skewed. Think about it: We hear stories about people dropping four hundred pounds, but how often do you really know how much body fat that person lost? If you look closely at some of the people on the Richard Simmons shows or on *The Biggest Loser*, you can still see a significant amount of body fat in particular areas.

When you drop weight too quickly, that's a problem, too. On the other hand, if you're training correctly, you'll typically lose weight at a pretty safe rate.

TYPES OF FAT

Your body has several types of fat. The main ones we need to talk about here are subcutaneous and visceral fat. Subcutaneous fat lies directly under your skin, and visceral fat is the fat around your organs.

SUBCUTANEOUS FAT

Subcutaneous fat is the kind you can pinch with your fingers. If you've ever had fat calipers used on you, that's the kind of fat that's being measured. Fat that covers your abdominal muscles is subcutaneous fat, which men and women tend to have in equal proportion. You can generally reduce your level of this as long as you have the right nutritional program; you don't lose subcutaneous fat with exercise as much as you do by eating properly. Again, this is one of the reasons that sit-ups won't give you six-pack abs by themselves; in order to see the definition, you have to strip off the fat, and the best way to do that is through diet.

VISCERAL FAT

Visceral fat is deeper inside your body, behind the abdominal wall. It surrounds internal organs and helps cushion the jostling they get when you move around. You don't want to bruise your intestines, so that fat is a good thing—up to a point. However, hormones secreted by visceral fat can cause all kinds of metabolic problems. They may prevent an appropriate insulin response and/or trigger inflammation.[6] I've had clients with swelling that was caused by visceral fat pushing outward on the abdominal walls.

The only way to lose visceral fat is through high-intensity work, preferably circuit training with weights.

Sprints are the best way to take care of visceral fat. Likewise, building muscle is vital to good health and maintaining a healthy, long-term body-fat percentage. The joke among good strength coaches is that programs focused only on losing weight turn really big fat people

Visceral fat, unlike subcutaneous fat, isn't primarily dictated by your diet, so the only way to take it off is through exercise—and that doesn't mean doing sit-ups.

into really little fat people. Take Tommy Lasorda. Even though he's a lot smaller, in my view he looks depleted. He's lost the muscle that would have kept the fat off. Every time he goes off his diet, he gets bigger and always will —unless he continues to starve himself and do cardiovascular work every single day of his life. What's more, his skin is going to just hang on him. No one wants to look like a lizard whose epidermis is three times too big for him.

You frequently see women in their fifties and sixties with a tremendous amount of loose skin hanging from their arms and other body parts. This is primarily because they have lost too much muscle. It's not pretty and it's not the way the body is supposed to look or function.

---

[6] Klein, S., et al. "Effect of Liposuction on Insulin Action and Coronary Heart Disease Risk Factors," *New England Journal of Medicine* 350: 2549-2557, 2004.

The thing is, you don't need to starve. You need to eat better so your body is more inclined to take off the fat and use it to build muscle. You should eat a well-rounded diet that includes some good fats as well as a lot of protein and some clean carbohydrates. Further, everybody should manage insulin levels by eating more frequently.

To summarize how you should exercise in order to lose fat, we advise the following:

❖ **Use strength training as seventy-five percent of your training protocol.**

When you lift weights, adding muscle and losing fat is about a one-to-one ratio.

❖ **If you're overweight, don't run**.

If you want to do some occasional cardio work, get on a bike, an elliptical, or a rowing machine.

❖ **Do interval training.**

After you warm up, go fast for a minute, then slow for a minute and a half—you can always increase your ratio of fast to slow after you get better conditioned. We've had a lot of success with our clients on interval training; the heart rate gets up a lot higher, and it's anaerobic in nature, so you're burning more fat while preserving muscle.

❖ **Take a walk.**

This is fine for anybody who is reasonably healthy with decent balance; it doesn't matter how overweight you are. If you only have access to flat ground, speed up and slow down by intervals, but ideally, you should walk up and down hills, which is a very natural kind of interval training. Negotiating natural obstacles is good training for moving your body through three dimensions and building a lot of different types of functional strength, because your activities are changing all the time.

LOSING FAT FOR THE OVER-FIFTY CROWD

According to common myth, losing weight gets trickier the older you get. Conventional wisdom says that as you age, you should use lighter weights, do a larger number of reps, and do more cardio work.

It's true that cardio work is harder on your joints as you get older, but using lighter weights simply means that it takes you longer to accomplish anything, from finishing your workouts to losing body fat. When you're just starting out with strength training, you may need to use lighter weights than someone who has been training for a long time, or than a twenty-year-old who has picked up a barbell for the first time. But that's just for starters.

Whether you're twenty or seventy years old, you need a program that addresses the imbalances in your body. You need to get a proper evaluation and find out whether you're leaning forward or to the side, whether one side of the body is stronger than the other, and so on. Regardless of age, your goal should be to get your body balanced and functioning so that your gait is steady when you walk, harnessing equal power from your hamstrings and quads.

Just because you're over fifty doesn't mean you have to lift less, as long as you're lifting smart and doing it in a professional program where you've assessed and addressed your body's imbalances.

You can still lift increasingly heavy weights over the years without injury, no matter how old you are. It's possible to be a much stronger person at sixty than you were at fifty.

I should be clear here that I'm not implying you're going to be able to try out for the Olympics or break world records, nor are you going to be doing four-hundred-pound power snatches over your head. But you'll be able to move more weight as you keep training, provided you have balance. There is no doubt that you can add muscle mass as you get older; you just have to work smarter in order to do so.

There are two types of muscle contractions: concentric and eccentric. In a *concentric* contraction, the muscle fibers contract in order to exert force. While you're lifting a weight in an *eccentric* contraction, the muscle fibers contract in order to keep a weight from going out of control while you're lowering it slowly.

If you're squatting, lunging, or otherwise lowering your body over a period of three seconds or longer, your muscles continue to contract via eccentric contractions. This is exactly what you want. Eccentric contractions aren't only good for training your muscles with both lifting and lowering, but they will also raise your metabolism. According to several studies, eccentric contractions are associated with increased calorie burn and muscle growth.[7]

> You don't need to work out for two to three hours a workout, over and over again, as you get older. Instead, with the help of a professional trainer, you can put together phenomenal programs that range from twenty to forty minutes, taking advantage of eccentric contractions to accomplish your goals with maximum efficiency.

So how do you exercise using eccentric contractions? With weights, because that's what you do naturally anyway. After about 35-45 minutes, most people have peaked in their ability to build muscle and burn fat. Once you get balanced, you don't need to add increased reps to your routines; you need *better* routines. (You can contact us through the Ageless Human website or at the Duffy Fitness Institute and ask about an evaluation for you or a loved one.)

Losing body fat isn't the only concern we have over fifty. There are four major mid-life concerns that strength training can help.

INCREASING TESTOSTERONE

As we get older, men's testosterone levels start to diminish, and in addition to maintaining sexual health, these levels have been shown to correlate with many of the parameters associated with a lower risk of cardiovascular disease, such as increased lean body mass, decreased visceral fat mass, decreased total cholesterol, and glycemic control.

---

[7] Hackney, Kyle J. et al. "Resting Energy Expenditure and Delayed-Onset Muscle Soreness After Full-Body Resistance Training With an Eccentric Concentration," *The Journal of Strength and Conditioning Research*, 22 (5), 1602-160.

There are two excellent and natural methods to increase and maintain your testosterone level: 1) Strength training; and 2) Diet.

Strength training increases your natural testosterone levels.[8] There's something about the intensity of the workout that accomplishes this. Even runners working at fifty-five percent of their bodies' VO_2 max levels don't see a testosterone increase as high as those doing strength training.

Your diet can also have a big effect. Eating soy products (which contain phytoestrogens) may lower your testosterone levels,[9] and drinking from BPA plastic bottles may do the same,[10] so you want to stay away from both.

RAISING METABOLIC RATES

As we get older, our metabolic rate decreases, but it's possible to maintain your rate through strength training. We talked about the fact that women of any age who don't strength train are at risk for metabolic syndrome. The same is true for anyone as they age for the same reason: low muscle mass.

If you want a good metabolism, add muscle mass. People with a high ratio of muscle to fat have a high metabolic rate.

People who work out via strength training can eat much more without gaining body fat than those who don't. If you're eating correctly, you're not feeding the fat, you're feeding the muscle. The amount you eat should be relative to the amount of muscle you have. When you have a lot of muscle, your body is more sensitive to overload and "tells" you how much to eat. Because your body is producing less cortisol, you'll have fewer food cravings.

---

[8] Tremblay, Mark S., et al. "Effect of Training Status and Exercise Mode on Endogenous Steroid Hormones in Men," *Journal of Applied Physiology*, 1988, 65:2406-2412.

[9] Weber, K.S., et al. "Dietary Soy-phytoestrogens Decrease Testosterone Levels and Prostate Weight without Altering LH, Prostate 5alpha-Reductase or Testicular Steroidogenic Acute Regulatory Peptide Levels in Adult Male Sprague-Dawley Rats," *Journal of Endocrinology*, September 1, 2001 170 591-599.

[10] Li, D., et al. "Occupational Exposure to Bisphenol-A (BPA) and the Risk of Self-Reported Male Sexual Dysfunction," *Human Reproduction* (2010) 25 (2): 519-527.

Not long ago, I ran into a woman at a jazz concert whose figure—from the back—resembled that of a thirty-year-old. When she turned around, her face revealed that she was in her late sixties or so, but the muscles in her legs and throughout her body were toned and her posture was perfect.

She shared that she didn't believe in the myths we're discussing in this book, and had actually done all the exercises that we teach—squats, lunges, and so on—over a long period of time. As a result, she maintained good, lean muscle tissue mass in her body and no doubt enjoyed a high metabolic rate.

INCREASING FLEXIBILITY

Many people over fifty have problems with decreased flexibility. Strength training can help with that, too; however, flexibility is only part of what you need to protect your joints. You may be the most flexible person in the world and still injure yourself if you don't focus on stabilizer muscles, too.

A good strength program will evaluate your flexibility and help you increase pliancy in areas you need in order to move with optimal functionality. Through strength training, you can become flexible enough to do a squat and strong enough to keep from wobbling.

> You don't need to be able to lock your feet behind your head in order to consider yourself flexible. You just need to have full range of motion.

In general, your joints will remain stronger if you strength train because you're working the stabilizers for those joints. This, in turn, prevents the primary muscles of the body from bending the joints improperly. People often end up with sore joints because their stabilizer muscles aren't strong enough to support their movement, not because they're not flexible enough.

Range-of-motion exercises relieve stiffness in general and help maintain your ability to keep what you have—as the saying goes, use it or lose it. When you add free weights to range-of-motion exercises, it's particularly good for you because you're strengthening your muscles, too. If you do a full-range lunge, squat, or bent-over row, you are using the optimum power and range of your joints.

Consider also exercising in an unstable position, because doing so fires up even more muscles as you work to keep your balance. This is one of the things I learned at the CHEK Institute. It worked very effectively on me personally, and I recommend similar exercises for our clients.

Building exercises around a Swiss ball destabilizes people. A Swiss ball is unstable in different directions—even up and down—so you are forced to connect the actions of your primary muscles with your stabilizers and neutralizers in order to keep your balance. From what I've seen at the DFI (and in my personal life), the habit of working all your muscles together facilitates joint stability and reduces your chance of injury.

We also recommend exercising using only one leg or arm, which forces the body to be balanced and makes sure that the small muscles are engaged to support the big muscles. This helps prevent joint pain and potential muscle tears. Being efficient and functional will keep your body toned, and you'll feel, look, and act younger.

IMPROVING BRAIN FUNCTION

There is growing evidence that the over-fifty crowd benefits greatly from strength training exercise to improve cognitive function. This new research compiled in different studies over the past ten years has found remarkable improvement in neuro-degeneration for those who are engaged in strength-training exercise protocols three times a week. We see the lights go on all the time with our clients who begin programs at fifty, sixty, seventy, and even eighty years and older. These people are balancing on Swiss balls, can lift significant weight, and their body and mind function well. They move with ease and are not in pain, handling everyday activities like reaching for a high jar on a shelf or bending down to pick up the dog. We witness improvements every day in this age group with regard to reaction time, coordination, and memory.

Bottom line, the most significant reason for the demise of Americans' health is our lack of muscle. Many of us have physical imbalances and are so weak that we can't get through life without help: escalators, higher toilets, and handrails are everywhere—all to make life "easier." What's more, we're enabling a further decline in health in our kids.

Let's work on fitness and functionality, not a grab-all term like "weight-loss," which is virtually meaningless when it comes to health.

If you wish to discover how fit and functional you are and/or take a fitness quiz, sign up for virtual training at www.ageless-human.com, or come into our physical facility at the Duffy Fitness Institute for an evaluation and training program.

CRITICAL TAKEAWAY

FAT LOSS IS THE TRUE STRATEGY BEHIND WEIGHT LOSS.

MYTH BUSTER IN MOTION

As soon as we shift our focus to *fat* loss, weight loss is a natural end result.

Fat-burning exercises are high-intensity exercises that elevate your heart rate and are guided with sets, tempo, and rest periods.

Here are some great ones:

- ❖ Swiss ball exercises
- ❖ Weightlifting for biceps, triceps, and abs
- ❖ Lunges that reinforce posture and leg strength
- ❖ Sprints
- ❖ Multipoint circuits with lower- and upper-body sequence patterns

When you engage in high-intensity exercising for short periods of time with the appropriate rest in between, you raise growth hormone and testosterone, which are two important anti-aging hormones. In contrast, when you perform low-intensity exercise over long periods of time, you *increase* oxidative stress, which ages you and *lowers* anti-aging hormones. What's more, high-intensity strength training will burn **fat** 24-36 hours after exercising, whereas low-intensity exercise will burn more **muscle** than fat during the same time period.

MYTH 7

EATING LOW-FAT, LOW-CARB FOODS AND LESS RED MEAT IS THE BEST DIET FOR OPTIMUM HEALTH

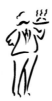

TRUTH:

Our bodies are designed to eat meat, vegetables, nuts, and fruits—frequently.

✗ Don't Starve Yourself:
How the body fights back

✗ Bad Calories:
Debunking the food pyramid

✗ Good Calories:
Never say "I'm sorry" again

✗ Vegetarianism:
Why initial results aren't sustained

Nutrition is a complex issue because our bodies are complex systems. Yet nutrition is logical and simple if we follow a clear, straightforward, and easy-to-remember program based on evolutionary principles, which I'll get to shortly.

The idea that simply eating less by cutting your calories is going to help you lose weight is a myth. But it has been drummed into us. If you tend to eat a lot of bad food—donuts and cupcakes and sugary foods—and then suddenly start eating less, sure, you're going see some benefits. However, if you never eat the food that's good for you, you won't get the nutrients you need to be healthy and mentally alert, and you won't reach your optimum body-fat percentage no matter how many workouts you do.

We need to start thinking of calories as "good calories" and "bad calories," just as we describe "good fats" and "bad fats." The plan should be to decrease the bad calories to clean out your system and stop the damage you're doing to yourself, and increase the good calories—though never to the point of feeling full.

DON'T STARVE YOURSELF

Regardless of what kind of calories you eat, you should never starve your body. You'll achieve the opposite result from what you intended.

Human beings as a species have physiological reactions built into our genes that help us survive. We call these survival instincts, and they go all the way down to the cellular and hormonal level.

Starvation means stress, and stress triggers your fight-or-flight system. As a result, your immune system is suppressed while your body focuses on fighting for calories. You can't lie to your body— mentally you might find ways not to feel hungry, but believe me, your body is still trying to fight the good fight.

And what is starving yourself going to do for you, anyway? As we saw earlier, if you're losing weight rather than reducing your body fat, you're destroying muscle and setting yourself up for future fat gain. You will enter a cycle of starvation, weight gain, starvation, weight gain … and so it will continue.

> You might think that by starving yourself, you're somehow going to lose weight—the less mass that comes in, the less mass you'll have in your body, right? But when you're starving yourself, your body assumes you can't get enough food, and so it holds onto fat and stores it for survival.

Many people assume that the body would burn fat first in survival mode, but it actually uses up muscle along with fat to ensure that it can carry out essential functions. Fat is a primary source of energy, but it doesn't contain all the nutrients necessary for survival, such as protein, so muscle breakdown also occurs.

Proteins are needed to create antibodies, contract muscles, and produce enzymes and hormones. If you're not getting protein, your body will literally cannibalize itself to get it. It doesn't matter how much fat, sugar, and starch you're consuming, your body will break down muscles and then store the excess calories as fat.

Your body needs both fat and muscle to survive.

You'll see some starvation victims, especially kids, whose bodies bloat up, even though their arms and legs are sticks.[11] They're getting some carbohydrates, but they're not getting any protein and their muscles get broken down. The swelling is caused by a combination of things: edema, or fluid build-up (especially in the feet and legs); visceral fat buildup in the abdomen, especially around the liver, which has to deal with all the waste materials of breaking down muscle tissue; and extra carbohydrates being converted to fat. You can't build protein tissue without protein.

You sometimes see the same thing with people who combine steady cardiovascular, aerobic work with a near-starvation diet. Those people are working against their bodies' primal functions, hard-coded in their DNA.

BAD CALORIES

Why do we get fatter on some calories than others? For two main reasons:

1. Eating food we can't digest
2. Eating poorly-raised food

FOOD WE CAN'T DIGEST

As far as nutrition goes, Americans have been sold a bill of goods. The focus on nutrition began in 1957 when the government released the publication

---

[11] This is called *kwashiorkor*, or "the sickness the baby gets when the new baby comes"—referring to weaning a toddler from milk and putting them on a low-protein diet.

"Essentials of an Adequate Diet" by Louise Page and Esther Hawley, which named four key food groups: meat, dairy, grains, and fruits and vegetables.

Then the food pyramid debuted in 1992. It was based on a similar food pyramid developed in 1974 by Anna Britt Agnsäter, head of the test kitchen for a Swedish retail/consumer cooperative. The pyramid was created in response to demands at that time for cheaper yet still nutritious food during food shortages in that country. From its base to the top, the 1992 pyramid suggested six to eleven servings of grains, three to five servings of vegetables, two to four servings of fruit, two to three servings of protein, two to three servings of dairy, and sparing use of oils and fats.

I often wonder how much damage that food pyramid did. It implied that eating a lot of grains was healthy. But that is not the case.

To see how the pyramid has evolved, visit our website at:
www.ageless-human.com

Many experts believe that as a species, we don't digest grains very well. It takes something like ten to twenty-five thousand years for the body to learn how to digest something new, and humans have only been eating grains for eleven thousand years at the most.[12] Most people in North America have been eating wheat for seven thousand years or less and corn for nine thousand years or less—and you know how well you digest corn kernels.

If you eat a lot of grains, it's easy to gain weight and bloat up. That's primarily due to a protein in some grains called gluten that causes problems for many people. In fact, about one percent of people in North America currently have Celiac disease, in which certain types of gluten cause the villi—or fingerlike projections in the small intestines that absorb nutrients—to separate and come off.[13]

> When you eat something that your body isn't able to digest well, the entire body reacts by swelling—adding fluid— to protect itself.

[12] We started with emmer, also known as farro, in the Fertile Crescent area of the Middle East. Interestingly, many people with moderate levels of gluten intolerance can eat emmer.

[13] Toman, Barbara. "Celiac Disease: On the Rise," *Discovery's Edge: Mayo Clinic's Online Research Magazine*, July 2010.

Some of the models I trained in the past were pudgy in their lower abdominal areas. They thought that leg lifts, crunches, and sit-ups would help them get rid of that fat. I ran food-allergy tests to determine whether they were allergic to anything, and in every single instance, the women with the extra fat experienced some kind of immune response to gluten or other elements. Once they stopped eating the foods that were causing immune responses—primarily breads, pasta, and rice—that pudginess disappeared.

POOR FOOD

Our food is being poorly cultivated. Here's why:

❖ Nutrition-depleted soil produces inferior crops.

❖ Many chemicals, including herbicides and pesticides, are added to our food supply during the production process.

❖ Food is being processed with lots of chemicals and hidden additives.

According to Charles Poliquin, about seven percent of the soil in this country is suitable for growing organic crops, which means about ninety-three percent is not. The rest of the soil is treated with all kinds of chemicals to ensure that enough food is produced to make a profit.

In America, we only spend about seven percent of our income on food. Globally, that's not a high percentage.[14] A person in China spends about thirty-three percent; in Pakistan, about forty-five percent. Even the French spend over thirteen percent on food. Americans are used to—and spoiled by—cheap food. Actually, we *insist* on cheap food, which by definition is raised cheaply, no matter how our bodies are affected.

We patronize fast-food restaurants instead of buying produce from organic grocery stores. We choose gas-station milk instead of going to farmers' markets. We love our junk food, and we have junk bodies to show for it.

---

[14] Jones, Natalie. "Mapping Global Food Spending (Infographic)," Civil Eats, March 29, 2011. http://civileats.com/2011/03/29/mapping-global-food-spending-infographic/ (accessed November 28, 2011).

THE ALLERGY EPIDEMIC

A myriad of studies show that the number of people with food allergies or intolerances is growing at a shocking rate, but professional medical practitioners and nutritional experts can't seem to agree on the cause.

In my opinion, people are eating things that (A) they haven't evolved to eat (such wheat and dairy), and (B) come from bad sources. This food is full of hormones, pesticides, and chemicals. And then, to top it off, we add more chemicals when we process the food. Naturally our bodies are going to react negatively. With so many drugs in our food, we're soon going to see drug interaction problems that make people's intolerances worse.

If you're eating clean—that is, food that you've evolved to eat and that hasn't been drugged up—it doesn't matter what kind of foods you mix together. We've progressed over time to eat everything obtainable to us when it's available.

GOOD CALORIES

The general consensus among most experts is that we're able to digest foods such as fruits and vegetables very well—and of course animal and other types of protein. If you stick to those types of calories, which I call the "good calories," I believe you can eat more or less whatever you want. In fact, a lot of people who are very healthy eat a substantial amount of food without putting on fat because they have a lot of muscle.

**You never want to eat until you feel full,
because at that point you're overeating.**

But if you're eating clean food, which means good sources of proteins (free range, wild, and organic, and no soybeans) and organic vegetables and fruits, you'll digest food quickly and easily. You won't feel bloated, either, which is pretty common in our culture right now.

Eating an adequate amount of good calories is the opposite of getting on the starvation/fat building cycle. You're informing your body that everything is okay—there is no starvation going on and no need to panic and store up calories.

Carrying around a lot of fat isn't good for you, and it puts a strain on your body. There are two reasons your body puts on fat:

❖ You've taught your body that it needs energy stores, no matter what the cost.

❖ You've overloaded your body with bad calories that it can't process properly.

Once you get rid of those problems, your body will adjust to its optimal weight, especially if you've built the muscle mass to maintain your metabolic rate at a high level.

PALEO DIET

So what's the simplest, easiest way to remember how to eat good calories? Only eat what your body has evolved to eat—by eating the way our long-ago ancestors did. I recommend the Paleo diet.

Our ancestors lived from about two-and-a-half million years ago to ten thousand years ago—before the age of agriculture. They were nomads who hunted and gathered. They mixed food types and ate everything they could get their hands on. They didn't eat bread, because there was no such thing as farming.

They hunted, and when they killed an animal, they lived on the carcass, eating it for breakfast, lunch, and dinner. They gathered fruits, vegetables, and nuts when they were ripe. All they ate, in other words, were animal proteins and unprocessed plants—the Paleo diet. In the same spirit, I believe you should eat all kinds of meat, fruits and vegetables, nuts, and seafood, in any kind of combination.

The Paleo Diet is basic, simple to understand, and makes logical sense. Most people who go on this kind of diet lose weight pretty quickly while putting on muscle at the same time. If it's true that it takes a long time for our digestive systems to adapt to new types of food, it makes sense to revert to what our digestive systems are proven to handle best.

For a sample day of a Paleo diet, visit our website at:
www.ageless-human.com

I know from personal experience with our clients that people who follow the Paleo diet have done remarkably well in achieving healthier bodies and increasing their fitness levels. Admittedly, it's tough to do in today's market because bad calories are generally inexpensive calories. If you want good, clean calories from grass-fed, free-range, or wild protein and from organically grown produce, you're going to have to seek it out and pay a premium.

Think about your priorities: If you eat bad calories, you're going to get fat and risk health issues. It's much cheaper to eat right in the first place than to treat health problems caused by a poor diet.

VEGETARIANISM

There are moral and other reasons why some people choose vegetarianism, and I understand that, but if you look at many who find vegetarianism beneficial, you'll discover that they're allergic to a number of things they're giving up. Often they've been eating bad animal proteins, so naturally they're going to feel better as they get rid of those toxins.

On the other hand, those same people are likely to face challenges in getting enough protein in their bodies without consuming the damaging hormones in soy, for example. They'll have issues obtaining vitamin B_{12}, which you can get from leafy greens (but not soy). It is so much simpler to get these vitamins from red meat, fish, poultry, dairy products, and eggs. A lot of vitamins and minerals are like that; you can get the vitamin directly from a plant-based source, but it's hard to get the levels you need without getting the vitamin from an animal that ate massive amounts of plants in the first place.

One of the greatest myths is that soy is a good replacement for animal protein. It isn't; unfortunately, the myth is everywhere.

Part of the fallout from not getting enough clean protein, and being short on essential vitamins and minerals, is that you potentially lose a tremendous amount of muscle in a brief period of time. Without that protein, your brain will not function efficiently.

Every health food store you visit—and even coffee houses, which are not about healthful food—has soy everything. Soy's cheap, and there's a lot of it, so it must be good for you, right?

But soy contains isoflavones, which act as antioxidants but may also mimic estrogens (i.e., they're phytoestrogens, or "plant-estrogens"). And these, eaten in large quantities, may reduce fertility in women, trigger premature puberty, and disrupt fetal and early-childhood development.[15]

Any doctor working in endocrinology will tell you that we have a true calamity today with the lack of testosterone on this planet. We have many young men coming of age who have lived on soy for long periods of time and now suffer estrogen issues, sometimes developing what we call "man boobs," not to mention that they have smaller testicles on average than they used to.

One reason for these changes is the large amount of soy in men's diets. You don't even have to eat tofu; soy is in everything now. If you go to a fast-food restaurant and order a hamburger, chances are you're getting soy in your bun (soy flour), soy in your meat (soy protein), and even soy in your sauces (soy sauce). And babies are getting more and more soy through their formula, too.

Now there are people from some cultures, Asians in particular, who digest soy well, because they've been eating it for thousands of years. In addition, the soy you get in Asia is not the same as the soy you get over here because they tend to raise their soy organically, avoiding a lot of problems. On the other hand, many Asian people have milk allergies, because they don't have the same history of drinking milk for thousands of years as people of Northern European descent do.

Bottom line: Stay away from soy, and make sure the animal protein you're eating is clean and healthful.

[15] Jefferson, W.N., et al. "Neonatal Exposure to Genistein Disrupts Ability of Female Mouse Reproductive Tract to Support Preimplantation Embryo Development and Implantation." *Biology of Reproduction*, March 2009, 80(3):425-431.

ANIMAL PROTEIN

It's vital to get animal protein in your diet. You can't feed people a one-hundred-percent carb diet and expect them to be healthy. Of course, bad animal protein doesn't do you much good either. The movie *Food, Inc.* very effectively points out the differences between grass-fed and corn-fed beef.

Cows have four compartments in their stomachs and regurgitate their food after it has been mixed with digestive juices to chew it further—and their digestive systems are adapted to process grass, not grains. These animals have only been domesticated for about ninety-five hundred years, and eating grains for less time than that. The fact that they have trouble digesting corn (and soy) diets is shown by the way their methane (gas) production drops almost twenty percent when they're raised on grass, rather than grains.[16]

With our increasing population over the centuries, there has been an increasing demand for food, and that's where the trouble started. During the last century, we had an abundance of grain (corn) and a demand for beef. The low-priced corn (and soy) grew in popularity as a crop because of the demand to use it as fodder for cows. Ranchers could raise cattle cheaper and more quickly feeding them grains. Of course, in order to keep those corn-fed cows healthy, we shoot them full of steroids and antibiotics. What's worse, they don't get to move around much—which as you know is not only inhumane, but is also not a recipe for building muscle tissue.

People who are eating corn-fed beef are eating drugged-up, unhealthy animals. You are what you eat; eating that kind of beef is bound to produce bad results.

Again, I understand why people go on vegetarian and vegan diets. They often get sick and decide that they can't digest meat—*any* meat. They certainly won't be able to if (A) they are consuming a bad source of beef, in particular, or (B) they eat an overall poor diet. The enzymes we need to break down food is largely contained in good-quality animal protein sources, and most people can eat grass-fed, hormone-free beef from a reputable farm with no dietary repercussions.

---

[16] Kaufman, Leslie. "Greening the Herds: A New Diet to Cap Gas," *The New York Times*, June 5, 2009. http://www.nytimes.com/2009/06/05/us/05cows.html (accessed November 28, 2011).

It's the same with chicken. Mass-production chicken ranches are simply appalling. If you get a free-range chicken that comes from a great farm and it isn't loaded with drugs after being trapped in a cage the size of a boom box, that chicken is a viable source of protein for you.

Likewise, eating wild-caught fish is important. In concentrated farming environments, we are feeding fish corn and soy, which is not a natural food source for the fish and the nutritional results are inconclusive. If you eat wild fish, you're going to have good, natural results.

We need protein to build muscle, maintain brain function, and produce enzymes and hormones within our bodies. In order to do this efficiently and in concert with the way we've evolved, we must start making better decisions about our protein sources.

We've gotten on the wrong track by rejecting all kinds of animal protein instead of making sure the animal protein that we do eat is good for us. Fortunately, there's a significant trend among farmers, ranchers, and consumers aimed at getting good food in front of people.

> Eggs are considered a perfect food, because they have lots of proteins and good fats that our bodies need.

While we're on the subject of food, let's talk about the egg-white myth. Our ancestors didn't track down eggs, crack them open, and then dump out the yolk, just eating the white. I'm certain they ate the whole egg. I believe the idea of only eating egg whites to keep your cholesterol down is a myth.

Charles Poliquin came onto my radio show and said that if you study eggs, you'll notice that nobody has actually proven that you will have cholesterol issues if you eat the whole egg. What happens is that some people with an allergy or intolerance for eggs have problems digesting them.

Most of the people I've trained tolerate eggs fine. I've loaded them up on eggs and watched their cholesterol go down. People may develop problems when they eat eggs (or any food, really) every day. If you eat certain foods too often and for too long, you're at more of a risk to develop an allergy to that food. If you switch up the foods you eat, you'll typically be fine. This, of course, mimics the hunting and gathering diet for which our bodies are hardwired.

SUPPLEMENTS

Sadly, the food we're eating, even if we eat clean, can't possibly contain the same nutritional content that it had ten thousand or even fifty years ago, because the soil isn't as rich with nutrients these days. That's why supplements are a must.

To guide you to better nutrition using supplements that effectively complement fitness programs, please carefully review our Notes on Nutrition section in the back of the book. Using these specially formulated supplements will maximize your physical and mental functionality.

If you start eating clean, good calories, and you get tested to see if you're consuming all the nutrients you need, it's probable that you're going to be low on certain vitamins or minerals, needing to supplement your diet with those nutrients that your body is missing.

One of the most glaring weaknesses we're seeing with crops raised in poor soil is that the foods that are produced lack enzymes. In the old days, food was abundant with enzymes that helped your digestive system break down the food. Now, because the food isn't quite up to par, you don't have access to the same enzymes. As a result, we're starting to see them in supplement form. Fortunately, taking enzymes is a short-term solution. After a while, your body naturally starts producing more of them on its own.

Nutrition is very challenging, especially now that food has become increasingly unhealthful through chemicals, hormones, and mass production.

The country's focus on nutrition is all about cheap, low-quality food.

Our outdated food pyramid made grains our largest source of calories, even though they don't provide proteins, vitamins, or minerals that we need —only calories (and a little dietary fiber).

My advice: Eat clean food—grown and prepared in traditional ways— despite the signals that our media, marketing, and culture send us. The more we demand food that is natural and clean, the more pressure there will be on the industry to produce healthy foods.

It may take a considerable amount of time and effort for our culture to cultivate food that will prevent health problems. Until then, make an investment in eating clean by choosing a Paleo-style diet. Not only will it produce terrific results for you almost immediately, but doing so will encourage the system to make those foods more accessible to you, your children, and your grandchildren.

CRITICAL TAKEAWAY

FAT IS NOT THE ENEMY; PROCESSED FOODS FILLED WITH SUGAR, GRAINS, AND CHEMICALS ARE WHAT'S CAUSING OUR RAPID DEMISE.

MYTH BUSTER IN MOTION

Fat, carbs, and red meat have been given a bad reputation. Americans are taught to believe that eating any or all makes you fat and causes disease when the opposite is actually true: fat is the missing nutrient in the American diet, good carbs are necessary for proper function, and organic animal protein provides vitamins that boost our health.

A Paleo Diet, in combination with high-quality supplements, is a nutritional plan that is highly effective for anti-aging. Provided you don't have any allergies to the following foods or problems digesting them, you should incorporate as many of these as possible into your everyday diet:

❖ Free-range, cruelty- and hormone-free poultry

❖ Grass fed, cruelty- and hormone-free beef

❖ Wild, not farm-raised seafood

❖ Organic fruits and vegetables

❖ Lots of organic greens

❖ A variety of nuts

❖ Free-range eggs

❖ Plenty of purified water

Please refer to our Notes on Nutrition and our website for a complete list of nutritional support, including recommended supplements at:
www.ageless-human.com

CONCLUSION

In America, we've been influenced to do exactly the wrong exercise programs and to eat food that is not good for our bodies. Why?

While I believe the people spreading these myths started out with good intentions, their information was built without scientific research and popularized by celebrities for a *marketing* advantage, not a *health* advantage.

There were economic reasons, too. Farmers saw the collapse of the prices of their crops at the same time that demand was going up, and they fought to save their income. They knew they weren't going to get paid for raising real food, so they grew what would make them any possible profit—grains. America is now the world's top producer of corn and the fourth largest grower of wheat.

The same thing happened with ranchers. Prices for corn dropped and expenses for raising cattle soared, so the logical solution was to feed them corn. Food became less nutritious, and people ate more and more to satisfy their appetites—until they started getting fat, and even obese.

As hundreds of millions of Americans eat poorer and poorer foods in larger and larger quantities, an epidemic of obesity has spread across the country. In order to lose that excess fat, we have to modify our diets to follow the blueprint for which our digestive systems were designed—the Paleo diet —and do exercises that come naturally to us, based on our evolutionary history. Yet we continue to see an increasing number of people turn to aerobic exercise and starvation diets to lose weight, no matter how short term that loss may be. These people become skinny and flabby, and then fat and flabby, and then skinny and flabby again, until they run out of strength to keep going and settle with simply being fat.

Because our metabolisms have been compromised by our bad choices, those of us who aren't eating right and exercising appropriately as we grow older will experience health problems from heart disease to diabetes. Also, our immune systems have become slaves to the pharmaceutical industry. It is easier to believe marketing messages that suggest we can be happier and more fit through medication without exercise than to engage in time-consuming exercises that tire us.

So here we are: bad food, a lack of knowledge about the best kinds of exercise to make us fit, and a plethora of so-called cures that are almost worse than the disease.

Our country is not figuratively, but *literally*, dying by degrees.

But we can turn things around. Here's how:

❖ We need true anti-aging programs that build muscle—for men and women of all ages—and that use efficient strength training for maximum functionality, improved cognition, and balanced hormones.

❖ We need a change in diet that focuses on good, clean calories, maintains a lean (and naturally attractive) body type, and promotes good health and longevity through the use of cutting-edge, high-grade nutritional supplements.

Imagine a country in which nobody was hungry and irritable; in which nobody had a bad back from extreme sit-ups or sparse muscle tissue; in which people didn't lack energy in the mornings; in which everybody had the nutrients they needed to make good decisions; in which all children had the right nutrition to build fit bodies and minds; in which being old didn't mean being practically helpless in a nursing home, but being fit, active, mentally alert, and looking good; in which being attractive didn't mean looking like a victim of starvation.

Every person who makes it a priority to build a healthy, fit lifestyle through exercise and nutrition makes it easier for everyone else in this country to succeed. As a social species, good, logical habits have the potential to become a preferred lifestyle, especially when positive, permanent results are openly and freely shared.

There's plenty of room for optimism. We are finally seeing people focus on building muscle tissue for their health—not just to grace the front covers of bodybuilding magazines. We see people making a point of eating organic, free-range, wild-caught, and grass-fed food. We see people turning away from aerobic exercise that tears their bodies up, and from soy products that irritate their systems and cause hormonal problems.

The megatrend toward life-logical exercise and nutrition has begun. We see it with the growth of awareness of organic foods and with public skepticism about big agribusiness. The word "gluten-free" is popping up on packaged foods, and the speed of information sharing continues to increase.

I want to work hard to show people how to maximize their benefits from exercising and eating right. But first we have to get the old myths out of the way. We need to clear out our legacy of bad health information and move toward a foundation of strength, fitness, longevity, function, and overall sound health based on ageless truths.

Keep the momentum going and share your success and knowledge with others. Join our community at www.ageless-human.com and together we can reverse the deadly trend that has plagued Americans, while reinstituting a foundation of health and fitness to ensure that our children and grandchildren thrive, and that we live to be fit, functional, and fabulous throughout our own lifetimes.

—Gordon Duffy

NOTES ON NUTRITION

Genes do not cast your destiny in stone, which explains the Ageless Human motto behind our supplements—*Beyond Genetics*.

Good nutrition and supplementation can offset gene weaknesses and enhance overall health and longevity, but the challenge is knowing what to buy that makes a real difference in achieving health goals.

Given the paucity of good, clean foods in this country—because of our poor soil and chemically-drenched animal and grain products—supplements are usually necessary for healthy living. A Paleo-style diet, in combination with our supplements and exercise protocols, truly provides the best recipe for good health.

Most of us are currently utilizing supplements as part of our health regimen, but the market is saturated. How do we know which brand is best combined with exercise and nutrition to reach our health goals? Which ones produce real results and increase our fitness and functionality for a lifetime?

Diabetes and obesity have reached epidemic proportions across the American population, and the numbers continue to rise every year. Many Americans think they are eating healthy and taking good supplements, but in reality they are raising their glucose and insulin levels, which directly affect the aging process.

At Ageless Human, our supplements are designed to maximize the synergies between functional exercise and clean nutrition to achieve long-term health.

FahBULOUS FISH OIL

This product carries the TruTG seal, guaranteeing that the fish oils are in their natural triglyceride form and are of unmatched TG potency. TG-bound omega-3 oils have a higher-than-industry standard for TG fish oil concentrate products with a potent 1400 mg of EPA/DHA. We have added Lipase as a digestive aid to promote better digestion of the fish oil and to reduce the incidence of a "fishy" aftertaste that is often experienced with other fish oils.

Fish oil has been shown to be very effective against the cellular inflammation caused by excessive daily exposure to omega-6 fats, sugars, and toxins. Also, the good fat from fish oil helps build and maintain muscle and aid in post-workout recovery. In addition, fish oil has been known to promote fat oxidation and improve insulin sensitivity as well as calorie partitioning.

ENHahNCED ENERGY

Mitochondria support of the cell is necessary as cells deteriorate with age and are exposed to free radicals. As mitochondria function declines, the cells become damaged and starved for energy, causing them to function inefficiently. Our formulary blend is designed to support efficient mitochondrial metabolism and energy (ATP) production. This product may be helpful for efficient fat burning, healthy weight loss, and improved overall cellular vitality and health.

ahPTIMUM ANTIOXIDANTS

We recommend this product as part of an overall health maintenance plan. This powerhouse antioxidant product presents a full-spectrum formula designed to help reduce the effects of oxidative stress and the production of free radicals.

DahGEST-IT ENZYMES and HCI SahPPORT

Every cell in your body needs enzymes for its biochemical functions, thus a deficiency will accelerate the aging process. As we age, our body's natural ability to produce optimum levels of stomach acid declines. These products were designed to aid the digestion process, thereby ensuring nutrients are properly absorbed.

METahBOLIC MULTIVITAMINS & MINERALS and CahMPLETE PROTEIN PLUS

Particularly vulnerable to oxidative stress are the Telomeres located at each end of our chromosomes. Telomere length has been proposed as a marker of biological aging. As DNA replicates, the telomere loses length. Shorter telomeres have been linked with higher mortality as well as an increased risk of chronic diseases. Epidemiological evidence exists that longer DNA telomere length is associated with multivitamin use. Therefore, in addition to adequate dietary protein, a good quality vitamin & mineral supplement is an effective anti-aging tool.

To improve physical and mental function, and for a younger and healthier YOU, be sure to consult our website for our complete list of supplements that support our fitness programs.

www.ageless-human.com

ACKNOWLEDGEMENTS

I would like to thank my fourth grade teacher, Mr. Flocco, who showed me my untapped potential; Mr. Dave Lucy who instilled my thirst for learning; and Sgt. Roberts, my drill instructor, who lived a real example of leadership.

Personally, I owe a heartfelt thanks to my three childhood friends: Michael, John, and Mark, who framed my foundation for friendship.

In the world of fitness and business, I extend my sincere gratitude to Paul Chek, Bill Pearl, and Charles Poliquin.

Big thanks go out to Chris and Janet, Ash, Len, Robert, and Steve who had the foresight to see my vision and offer their support of bringing this vision to you.

Thanks to my sisters, Jean and Betty, and to my brothers Alec, Richard, and my departed brother Jim. Thanks to my Dad, who taught me about food, and to my mother who, at 99, was a mental giant. And Karen, my driving force and love.

To all of my incredible friends and clients who have believed in my scientific method of fitness and health.

And finally, thanks to my dedicated and loyal team including Cynthia, Ronni, John, Matt, Phil, and Gary.

And of course, thanks go to Millie, who in high school told me I couldn't wear a tank top.

RESOURCES

The following books and articles (in print and online) may be helpful to you in researching various issues in this book:

Bittman, Mark. *Food Matters: A Guide to Conscious Eating, with More Than 75 Recipes*. New York: Simon & Schuster, 2009.

Bompa, Tudor O. and Gregory Haff. *Periodization*, Fifth Edition. Champaigne, IL: Human Kinetics, 2009.

Bompa, Tudor, Mauro Di Pasquale, and Lorenzo Cornacchia. *Serious Strength Training*, Second Edition. Champaigne, IL: Human Kinetics, 2003.

CHEK Institute, The. *CHEK Institute with ptEnhance*[TM]*: Implementing the Art and Science of Performance & Wellbeing*, 2011. http://www.chekinstitute.com/ (accessed December 16, 2011).

Daniel, Kayla T., PhD, CCN. *The Whole Soy Story: The Dark Side of America's Favorite Health Food*. Washington, DC: New Trends Publishing, Inc., 2005.

Diamond, Jared. *Guns, Germs, and Steel: The Fates of Human Societies*. New York: W. W. Norton & Company, 1997.

Gladwell, Malcolm. *Outliers: The Story of Success*. New York: Little, Brown and Company, 2008.

Hackney, Kyle J., Hermann-J Engels, and Randall J. Gretebeck. "Resting Energy Expenditure and Delayed-Onset Muscle Soreness After Full-Body Resistance Training With an Eccentric Concentration," *The Journal of Strength and Conditioning Research*, 22 (5), 1602-160.

International Sports Science Association. *International Sports Science Association*, 2011. http://www.issaonline.com/ (accessed December 16, 2011).

Jefferson, W.N., E. Padilla-Banks, E.H. Goulding, S.C. Lao, R.R. Newbold, and C.J. Williams. "Neonatal Exposure to Genistein Disrupts Ability of Female Mouse Reproductive Tract to Support Preimplantation Embryo Development and Implantation," *Biology of Reproduction*, March 2009, 80(3): 425-431.

Jenner, P. "Oxidative Stress in Parkinson's Disease," *The Annals of Neurology*, 2003;53 Suppl 3:S26-36; discussion S36-8.

Jones, Natalie. "Mapping Global Food Spending (Infographic)," *Civil Eats*, March 29, 2011. http://civileats.com/2011/03/29/mapping-global-food-spending-infographic/ (accessed November 28, 2011).

Kaufman, Leslie. "Greening the Herds: A New Diet to Cap Gas," The *New York Times*, June 5, 2009. http://www.nytimes.com/2009/06/05/us/05cows.html (accessed November 28, 2011).

Klein, S., L. Fontana, V.L. Young, A.R. Coggan, C. Kilo, B.W. Patterson, and B.S. Mohammed. "Effect of Liposuction on Insulin Action and Coronary Heart Disease Risk Factors," *New England Journal of Medicine* 350: 2549-2557, 2004.

Knab, Amy M., Andrew R. Shanley, Karen Corbin, Fuxia Jin, Wei Sha, and David C. Nieman, FACSM. "A 45-minute Vigorous Exercise Bout Increases Metabolic Rate for 19 hours," *Medicine & Science in Sports & Exercise*: May 2011, Volume 43, Issue 5, p. 266.

Leeuwenburgh, C. and J. W. Heinecke. "Oxidative Stress and Antioxidants in Exercise," *Current Medical Chemistry* 2001, 8, 829-838.

Li, D., Z. Zhou, D. Qing, Y. He, T. Wu, M. Miao, J. Wang, X. Weng, J.R. Ferber, L.J. Herrinton, Q. Zhu, E. Gao, H. Checkoway, and W. Yuan. "Occupational Exposure to Bisphenol-A (BPA) and the Risk of Self-Reported Male Sexual Dysfunction," *Human Reproduction* (2010) 25 (2): 519-527.

Liu-Ambrose, Theresa, Ph.D., PT; Lindsay S. Nagamatsu, MA; Peter Graf, PhD; B. Lynn Beattie, MD; Maureen C. Ashe, PhD, PT; Todd C. Handy, PhD. "Resistance Training and Executive Functions," *The Archives of Internal Medicine* 2010; 170 (2): 170-178.

Ogden, Cynthia L., PhD, and Margaret D. Carroll, MSPH, Division of Health and Nutrition Examination Survey, *Prevalence of Overweight, Obesity, and Extreme Obesity Among Adults: United States, Trends 1960–1962 Through 2007–2008*. Washington, DC: Government Printing Office, 2010.

Page, Louise, and Esther F. Phipard. "Essentials of an Adequate Diet," *U.S. Dept. of Agriculture Home Economics Research Report, No. 3*. Washington: US GPO, 1957.

Poliquin, Inc. *Poliquin: World Leader in Strength & Health Education*, 2011. http://www.charlespoliquin.com/ (accessed December 16, 2011).

Pollan, Michael. *The Omnivore's Dilemma: A Natural History of Four Meals*. New York: The Penguin Press, 2006.

President's Council on Fitness, Sports, & Nutrition, The. *The President's Challenge*, 2011. http://www.presidentschallenge.org/ (accessed November 15, 2011).

Roach, Randy. *Muscle, Smoke & Mirrors, Vol. I & II*. Bloomington, IN: AuthorHouse, 2008.

Stein, Jeannine. "Strength Training Does More Than Bulk up Muscles," *Los Angeles Times*, February 13, 2011.

Toman, Barbara. "Celiac Disease: On the Rise," *Discovery's Edge: Mayo Clinic's Online Research Magazine*, July 2010.

Tremblay, Mark S., Jennifer L. Copeland, and Walter Van Helder. "Effect of Training Status and Exercise Mode on Endogenous Steroid Hormones in Men," *Journal of Applied Physiology*, 1988, 65:2406-2412.

Weber, K.S., K.D. Setchell, D.M. Stocco, and E.D. Lephart. "Dietary Soy-phytoestrogens Decrease Testosterone Levels and Prostate Weight without Altering LH, Prostate 5alpha-Reductase or Testicular Steroidogenic Acute Regulatory Peptide Levels in Adult Male Sprague-Dawley Rats," *Journal of Endocrinology*, September 1, 2001 170 591-599.

Wilson, James L., ND, DC, PhD *Adrenal Fatigue: The 21st Century Stress Syndrome*. Petaluma, CA: Smart Publications, 2001.

Zohary, Daniel, and Maria Hopf. *Domestication of Plants in the Old World: The Origin and Spread of Cultivated Plants in West Asia, Europe, and the Nile Valley*. Oxford, U.K.: Oxford University Press, 2000.

ABOUT THE AUTHOR

7 Exercise Myths That Are Killing Americans is Gordon Duffy's wakeup call to the world. As the founder of the Duffy Fitness Institute, he is dedicated to helping clients achieve optimal health through the utilization of scientifically based exercise methodology. He has trained over 400 amateur and professional athletes as well as business professionals, seniors, cancer patients, and the neurologically challenged, including those afflicted with ALS and Parkinson's Disease.

In addition, Gordon is the CEO of Ageless Human, LLC, a company that focuses on anti-aging solutions to increase the functional living of people worldwide. He is the national anti-aging expert in Canada and has launched a functional longevity program internationally with the prestigious Vistage International Group. He has also been retained to direct the Sports Medicine Department of the World Anti-Aging Optimal Healthcare facility in Shanghai, China.

Gordon holds a Master of Fitness Sciences degree from the International Sports Science Association (ISSA) in Hartford, CT. He is recognized by the renowned Poliquin Institute as a Certified Strength & Conditioning Specialist and is a graduate of CHEK Institute as a Corrective Holistic Exercise Kinesiologist. He is also the recipient of the Army commendation Medal of Honor.

ABOUT AGELESS HUMAN, LLC
AND
THE DUFFY FITNESS INSTITUTE

We offer the following comprehensive programs, products, and services:

PROGRAMS

- ❖ Individual In-House or Virtual Anti-Aging Fitness Programs
- ❖ Corporate Wellness Programs
- ❖ Youth Fitness Programs & Clinics
- ❖ Strength & Conditioning Programs for Specific Athletic Programs
- ❖ Become a Wall Street Athlete (designed for the busy executive)

SUPPLEMENTS

A high-quality line of Ageless Human private label nutritional supplements —"Daily Essentials" and "For Convenience" items—specifically chosen to support our anti-aging protocols. To provide optimal results, this "clean" line of products is manufactured to be free of potentially harmful ingredients commonly found in other supplements, such as gluten, fructose, artificial sweeteners, and soy protein.

PRESENTATIONS

Gordon Duffy and our highly trained staff are available for presentations for corporate events, specialty groups, and organizations.

EVALUATIONS

We highly recommend a complete body analysis before beginning any exercise program. Ideally, an evaluation is performed to determine structure, stability, and alignment of the body before we customize a prescription for fitness. To avoid injury, pain, and poor biomechanics, we design a program to increase good muscle recruitment where the body is working more efficiently and ergonomically. We review posture health and an overall anti-aging exercise strategy that optimizes health goals for function and longevity.

People visit us from all over the world to strategically ignite anti-aging fitness plans that promote long-term health benefits. We have the capability to virtually train those who are not local to us but would like to take advantage of our expertise in setting realistic fitness goals that promote life-changing results.

We are conveniently located near the Orange County John Wayne Airport in Irvine, California.

AGELESS HUMAN, LLC
THE DUFFY FITNESS INSTITUTE

Gordon W. Duffy, Founder
Corrective High Performance Kinesiologist, MFS, CSCS

17891 Sky Park Circle, Suites F & G
Irvine, CA 92614

Office: (949) 861-4183
Fax: (949) 861-4186
Toll Free: (888) 654-3486

email: gordonduffy@duffyfitness.com

www.ageless-human.com
www.duffyfitness.com